ON BEING ILL
BY VIRGINIA WOOLF

Introduction by Hermione Lee

with

NOTES FROM SICK ROOMS

BY JULIA STEPHEN

Introduction by Mark Hussey
Afterword by Rita Charon

D0879043

Paris Press
Ashfield, Massachusetts
2012

Library of Congress Cataloging-in-Publication Data

Woolf, Virginia, 1882-1941.
On being ill / by Virginia Woolf ; with Notes from sick rooms by
Julia Stephen ; introduction by Hermione Lee and Mark Hussey ;
afterword by Rita Charon, MD.
p. cm.
ISBN 978-1-930464-13-1 (pbk. : alk. paper)
1. Woolf, Virginia, 1882-1941--Health. 2. Diseases--Psychological
aspects. 3. Sick in literature. 4. Sick--Psychology. I. Lee, Hermione. II.
Hussey, Mark, 1956- . III. Charon, Rita. IV. Stephen, Julia Prinsep,
1846-1895. Notes from sick rooms. V. Title.
PR6045.O72O5 2012
823'.912—dc23
[B]

2012031389

978-1-930464-13-1

2 4 6 8 0 9 7 5 3 1

Printed in the United States of America.

ON BEING ILL

with

NOTES FROM SICK ROOMS

ON BEING ILL

with

NOTES FROM SICK ROOMS

PUBLISHER'S NOTE

IT IS WITH tremendous pride that Paris Press brings our 10th Anniversary Edition of *On Being Ill* into print with *Notes from Sick Rooms* by Julia Stephen, originally published in 1883. Combining the voices of daughter and mother in the body of this book is truly thrilling. It offers a unique textual conversation between patient (Virginia) and care giver (Julia) and invites a new understanding of Virginia Woolf's writing and life through this little-known book by Julia Stephen. Presenting both texts together also provides a useful guide for care givers and individuals in the medical field to accompany Virginia Woolf's extraordinary essay about the transformational effects of illness in a world that often pushes this universal experience deep into the shadows.

Reading these very different books side by side imparts a thread of intimacy that I am sure neither Virginia nor Julia would have imagined in their hours of writing. Echoes between *On Being Ill* and *Notes from Sick Rooms* in subject and tone present an interior family resemblance that mirrors the uncanny similarities of their physical appearance. The texts' proximity also suggests a source for the maternal longing that Woolf expresses in her writing.

In this new edition, Hermione Lee's original, expansive essay about *On Being Ill* and the life and work of Virginia Woolf appears intact and is as poignant as it was a decade ago. Mark Hussey's Introduction to *Notes from Sick Rooms* offers profound observations of the world of illness that both Julia and Virginia inhabited, and presents Virginia Woolf, her publications, and *On Being Ill* in the context of Julia Stephen's life and writing. Concluding this edition is an Afterword by Rita Charon, physician, scholar, and founder and director of Columbia University's Program in Narrative Medicine. Readers might happily begin the book at the end, or start it here, at the beginning. The Afterword crystallizes elements from *On Being Ill* and *Notes from Sick Rooms*, examining the texts as literary works as well as expressions that reflect the broader experience of patient and medical practitioner.

Paris Press offers deepest thanks to the Estate of Virginia Woolf and the Society of Authors as the Literary Representative for permission to publish this long-neglected essay. We owe immense thanks to Henrietta Garnett and the Estate of Vanessa Bell for permission to reproduce Vanessa Bell's original 1930 cover art from The Hogarth Press publication of this work. Thank you Karen Kukil for assistance with both editions, and for the inspiring conversation that sparked the research that led to the original publication of *On Being Ill*. We offer gratitude to the memory of Marc Comras, to Eva Schocken, Margery Adams, Emily Wojcik, Hans Teensma, Anne Leiby, Janlori Goldman, Linda Weidemann, the Massachusetts Cultural Council, and the generous supporters, interns, volunteers, and assistants who made the publication of this book possible. Special thanks to Michael Russem and Claudia Cohen for the letterpress, hand-bound limited edition of *On Being Ill* (available through Paris Press), and to the Mortimer Rare Book Room at Smith College.

I am indebted to Mark Hussey for making me aware of Julia Stephen's *Notes from Sick Rooms* and to Janlori Goldman for strongly urging Paris Press to include this text in the new edition. Immense thanks to Hermione Lee, Mark Hussey, and Rita Charon for their contributions to this edition, and special thanks to Michele Wick and Janlori Goldman for the online Study and Reader's Guides that accompany this book at www.parispress.org. Gratitude to Don Joint for his thoughtful and beautiful cover-art collage, which refers to Virginia Woolf's life and to Vanessa Bell's original cover art for *On Being Ill*.

When I first read *On Being Ill*, it resonated fiercely on a personal front. In the months that followed, I found myself in numerous conversations with people in the midst of common as well as acute illnesses. The same has happened with *Notes from Sick Rooms*. Julia Stephen's useful and detailed instructions on caring for the sick have proved immensely helpful when visiting friends who are critically ill. The marked exceptions are in the "Food" and "Remedies" sections, which include information specific for treating illness during the late 19th century, and should *not* be attempted today.

Paris Press dedicates this 10th Anniversary Edition to Eleanor Lazarus. It is my hope and the hope of Paris Press that Virginia Woolf's profound observations, along with the guidance of her mother, Julia Stephen, will offer comfort and affirmation to all people experiencing the transformations induced by illness while "the army of the upright" marches healthily by.

JAN FREEMAN
AUGUST 25, 2012

ON BEING ILL

INTRODUCTION

ON BEING ILL, one of Virginia Woolf's most daring, strange, and original essays, has more subjects than its title suggests. Like the clouds which its sick watcher, "lying recumbent," sees changing shapes and ringing curtains up and down, this is a shape-changing essay, unpredictably metamorphosing through different performances. It "treats" not only illness, but language, religion, sympathy, solitude, and reading. Close to its surface are thoughts on madness, suicide, and the afterlife. For good measure, it throws in dentists, American literature, electricity, an organ grinder and a giant tortoise, the cinema, the coming ice age, worms, snakes and mice, Chinese readers of Shakespeare, housemaids' brooms swimming down the River Solent, and the entire life-story of the third Marchioness of Waterford. And, hiding behind the essay, is a love-affair, a literary quarrel, and a great novel in the making. This net or web (one of the key images here) of subjects comes together in an essay which is at once autobiography, social satire, literary analysis, and an experiment in image-making. By its sleight-of-hand and playfulness, and its appearance of having all the "space and leisure" in the world for allusion and deviation, it gallantly makes light of dark and painful experiences.

Illness is one of the main stories of Virginia Woolf's life.[1] The breakdowns and suicide attempts in her early years, which can be read as evidence of manic depression (though that diagnosis has also been hotly contested) led, in the thirty years of her adult writing life, to persistent, periodical illnesses, in which mental and physical symptoms seemed inextricably entwined. In her fictional versions of illness, there is an overlap between her accounts of the delirium of raging fever (Rachel in *The Voyage Out*), the terrors of deep depression (Rhoda in *The Waves*), and the hallucinations and euphoria of suicidal mania (Septimus in *Mrs. Dalloway*). All her life, severe physical symptoms—fevers, faints, headaches, jumping pulse, insomnia—signalled and accompanied phases of agitation or depression. In her most severe phases, she hardly ate, and shed weight frighteningly. Terrible headaches marked the onset of illness or exhaustion. The link she makes in the essay between "fever" and "melancholia" was

well known to her. Her jumping pulse and high
temperatures, which could last for weeks, were
diagnosed as "influenza"; in 1923, the presence of
"pneumonia microbes" was detected. At the beginning of 1922, these symptoms got so bad that she
consulted a heart specialist who diagnosed a "tired"
heart or heart murmur. Teeth-pulling (unbeliev-
ably) was recommended as a cure for persistent high
temperature—and also for "neurasthenia." (So the
visit to the dentist in *On Being Ill* is not a change of
subject.) It seems possible, though unprovable, that
she might have had some chronic febrile or tubercu-
lar illness. It may also be possible that the drugs she
was taking, for both her physical and mental symptoms, exacerbated her poor health. "That mighty
Prince" "Chloral" is one of the ruling powers in
On Being Ill. (The other, less sinister, presiding
deities—as opposed to the God of the Bishops—are
"Wisest Fate" and "Nature.") Chloral was one of
the sedatives she was regularly given, alongside dig-
italis and veronal, sometimes mixed with potassium
bromide—which could have affected her mental
state adversely. With the drugs went a regime of
restraint: avoidance of "over-excitement," rest cures,
milk and meat diets, no work allowed. All her life,

she had to do battle with tormenting, terrifying
mental states, agonising and debilitating physical
symptoms, and infuriating restrictions. But, in her
writings about illness—as here—there is also a
repeated emphasis on its creative and liberating
effects. "I believe these illnesses are in my case—
how shall I express it?—partly mystical. Something
happens in my mind."[2] *On Being Ill* tracks that
"something" in the "undiscovered countries," the
"virgin forest," of the experience of the solitary
invalid.

The immediate story behind the writing of *On
Being Ill* begins with Virginia Woolf falling down in
a faint at a party at her sister's house in Charleston
on August 19th, 1925. The summer had been
going swimmingly up till then. *Mrs. Dalloway* and
The Common Reader were published earlier in the
year, and whenever she "registered" her books'
"temperature" they seemed to be doing well. She
was full of ideas for starting her next novel, *To the
Lighthouse*, and she was at the most intimate stage
of her absorbing, seductive relationship with Vita
Sackville-West. But then, "why couldn't I see or
feel that all this time I was getting a little used up
& riding on a flat tire?"[3] The faint led to months

and months of illness, and her letters and diary, from September till the New Year (when no sooner did she start to get better than she contracted German measles) are full of frustration and distress. "Have lain about here, in that odd amphibious life of headache…" "I cant talk yet without getting these infernal pains in my head, or astonishingly incongruous dreams." "I am writing this partly to test my poor bunch of nerves at the back of my neck…." "Comatose with headaches. Cant write (with a whole novel in my head too—its damnable)." "The Dr has sent me to bed: all writing forbidden." "Can't make the Dr. say when I can get up, when go away, or anything." "I feel as if a vulture sat on a bough above my head, threatening to descend and peck at my spine, but by blandishments I turn him into a kind red cock." "Not very happy; too much discomfort; sickness…a good deal of rat-gnawing at the back of my head; one or two terrors; then the tiredness of the body—it lay like a workman's coat."[4]

During these slow months, two friendships were changing shape. Vita Sackville-West was tender and affectionate to Virginia Woolf in her illness, and making herself more valuable by the threat of absence: her husband, Harold Nicolson, was being posted by the Foreign Office to Persia; Vita would be off, from Kent to Teheran. (The 1926 version of *On Being Ill* made a private joke—later cut out—about how, in an imaginary heaven, we can choose to live quite different lives, "in Teheran and Tunbridge Wells.") Their letters became more intimate, and Woolf noted in her diary that "The best of these illnesses is that they loosen the earth about the roots. They make changes. People express their affection."[5] Just so, in *On Being Ill*, "illness often takes on the disguise of love..." wreathing "the faces of the absent...with a new significance" and creating "a childish outspokenness." That longing for the absent loved one, and the desire to call out for her, would make its way into *To the Lighthouse*. *On Being Ill* anticipates the novel in other ways too: her joke about the mind in its "philosopher's turret" prepares for Mr. Ramsay, and the essay's frequent images of water, waves, and sea-journeys spill over into the novel. In illness, she says in the essay, "the whole landscape of life lies remote and fair, like the shore seen from a ship far out at sea." Cam, in the boat going to the lighthouse, will echo this: "All looked distant and peaceful and strange. The shore seemed refined, far away, unreal. Already the little distance they had sailed had put them far from it and given it the changed look, the composed look, of something receding in which one has no longer any part." Absence and distance are themes in both essay and novel.

The other changing friendship of 1925 was more of an irritant; but the essay would not have been written without it. In the 1920's, the Woolfs and their Hogarth Press had become closely involved with T. S. Eliot. They published his *Poems* in 1919 and *The Waste Land* in 1922; he published a story of Woolf's in his magazine, the *Criterion*, also in 1922. He praised, and published, her essay "Character in Fiction" in 1924; The Hogarth Press published his essays on Dryden, Marvell, and the Metaphysical Poets alongside her essay "Mr. Bennett and Mrs. Brown" in the Hogarth Essays; and she tried to help him to the literary editorship of the *Nation* (which in the end Leonard Woolf took on instead). All this literary reciprocity and mutual assistance ran into difficulties when Eliot, in 1925, became a rival publisher at Faber & Gwyer, stole one of the Woolfs' authors, and reprinted *The Waste Land* without warning them. "Tom has treated us scurvily."[6] It was the beginning of her frequent criticisms of him for slyness, ruthlessness, and creepy egotism. And it was a difficult moment for him to be commissioning an essay from her for his revamped *New Criterion*, an invitation which she accepted in flattering terms ("Of course I should think it an honour to figure in your first number")[7] but was late in sending ("Dear Sir," she wrote half-jokingly, "I am sending my essay tomorrow, Saturday morning, so that I hope it will reach you in time. I am sorry to have delayed, but I have been working under difficulties").[8] His response to *On Being Ill* was unenthusiastic, and, characteristically, this threw her into a state of depression and anxiety: "I saw wordiness, feebleness, & all the vices in it. This increases my distaste for my own writing, & dejection at the thought of beginning another novel."[9] Does Lily Briscoe's anger at Charles Tansley's criticism in *To the Lighthouse* ("Women can't paint, can't write") partly find its inspiration here?

Eliot's publication of *On Being Ill* in the *New Criterion* for January 1926 was the first of several outings for the essay. It took its place here in a highminded quarterly publication which Eliot said, in his preface ("The Idea of a Literary Review") to the first issue, was intended to be "an organ of documentation" of "the development of the keenest sensibility and the clearest thought of ten years," formed on "the interests of any intelligent person with literary taste."[10] *On Being Ill* rubbed shoulders with a story by Aldous Huxley, an instalment of Lawrence's "The Woman Who Rode Away," a baffling piece of Gertrude Stein's ("The Fifteenth of November"), an essay by Cocteau, a reminiscence of Oscar Wilde by Ada Leverson, reviews of the latest arts news in London, Europe, and New York, a round up of foreign quarterlies, and analytical pieces on subjects such as "Aristotle on Democracy and Socialism."

Friends praised *On Being Ill*, and Leonard particularly admired it. The Woolfs made sure that the essay had a life outside Eliot's pages. As a result, it has gone through as many shape-shifts as the clouds it describes. In April 1926, a shortened version was published in a New York magazine (edited by Henry Goddard Leach), *The Forum*, under the title "Illness: An Unexploited Mine." This was a much more glossy, middle-brow setting, with many more "issues" under discussion ("Is Democracy Doomed?

A Debate"; "A Plea for Psychical Research"; "Farming the Ocean"; "The Problem of Anti-Semitism"), some rousing documentaries ("Horse Bandits and Opium"; "To the North Pole by Air-ship" by Fridjof Nansen), illustrations, and light fiction ("And No Questions Asked!" a short story by Viola Paradise, all in dialogue). Contributors were introduced with brief biographical notes, called "Toasts": "From the appearance of her first book...Mrs. Woolf has been the centre of great literary interest...Gradually the public has followed the lead of the critics, and her latest novel, *Mrs. Dalloway*, was widely acclaimed...The little essay with which she makes her debut in *The Forum* reveals her in a quietly contemplative mood."[11] This version of *On Being Ill* ended with the remark about the Chinese readers of *Antony and Cleopatra*, and cut the last passages on Shakespeare and Hare.[12]

In July 1930, Virginia Woolf typeset a new edition of 250 copies of *On Being Ill* for a Hogarth Press pamphlet. She signed each copy, exaggerating in her diary the labour of sitting in front of "the handmade paper on wh. I have to sign my name 600 times."[13] Vanessa Bell designed an appealing new

jacket. It was an attractive publication, if not a perfect one, as this mock-apology of Woolf's, written
in case of criticism, but not sent, makes clear:

> As one of the guilty parties I bow to your stric-
> tures upon the printing of On Being Ill. I agree that
> the colour is uneven, the letters not always clear,
> the spacing inaccurate, and the word 'campion'
> should read 'companion'.
>
> All I have to urge in excuse is that printing is a
> hobby carried on in the basement of a London
> house; that as amateurs all instruction in the art
> was denied us; that we have picked up what we
> know for ourselves; and that we practise printing in
> the intervals of lives that are otherwise engaged. In
> spite of all this, I believe that you can already sell
> your copy for more than the guinea you gave, as the
> edition is largely over subscribed, so that though
> we have not satisfied your taste, we hope that we
> have not robbed your purse.[14]

For this edition, Woolf made all kinds of small
changes from the 1926 *New Criterion* version. She
cut a mocking passage, from the section on
the Bishop and the believers, about the need for the
Bishop to have a new motor car—"but this Heaven

making needs no motor cars; it needs time and con-
centration"—perhaps because it felt out-of-date. She
tinkered considerably, too, with the wording about
lines of poetry which speak to us in illness, cutting
phrases about words which "spread their bright
wings, swim like coloured fish in green waters,"
words which "ripple like leaves, and chequer us
with light and shadow." It's as if, on re-reading, this
eloquent, mysterious passage seemed too fanciful to
her. Most revealingly, she cut a whole section in the
passage about reading Shakespeare without intermediaries, on how re-reading *Hamlet* is to re-read
one's own youth: "Thus forced always to look back
or sidelong at his own past the critic sees something
moving or vanishing in *Hamlet*, as in a glass one sees
the reflection of oneself." This, she may have felt,
was too self-revealing to keep.

After Virginia Woolf's death, Leonard Woolf
reprinted the 1930 version of the essay twice, once
in *The Moment and Other Essays* (1947) and again in
the fourth volume of *Collected Essays* (1967), where
he inaccurately gave its first publication date as
1930, perhaps as a way of wiping out Eliot's earlier
connection to the essay altogether. Since then, the
successive versions of the essay are being reprinted

in Andrew McNeillie's edition of Virginia Woolf's
essays. That this magnificent, fully annotated edition only began publication in 1986 is a mark of
how complicated and mixed the posthumous life of
Woolf's essays has been. It has taken a long time for
them to be read for their own sake, and for attention
to be paid to their literary strategies and thought-
processes.[15] Recent critical readings of the essays'
tactics of apparent looseness and spontaneity, of
interruptive open-endedness and refusal of authority, have looked especially closely at those which
refuse categorisation and slip across and between
genres—not manifesto, or literary criticism, or
feminist argument, or meditation on life, or fiction
or biography or history or autobiography, but a
curious, original mixture of all these: essays such
as "Street Haunting," "Thunder at Wembley,"
"Evening Over Sussex," "Hours in a Library,"
"On Not Knowing Greek," "The Sun and the
Fish," "How Should One Read a Book?"—and
On Being Ill. And this essay has, in recent years,
gained another kind of recognition in a burgeoning
literature of pathology, cited on medical websites
alongside books like Anne Hawkins's *Reconstruct-
ing Illness: Studies in Pathography* (1993), Arthur

Frank's *The Wounded Storyteller: Body*, *Illness*, *and
Ethics* (1995), Thomas Couser's *Recovering Bodies:
Illness, Disability, and Life Writing* (1997), and
Oliver Sacks's *A Leg to Stand On* (1994).

Eliot's lukewarm reception of *On Being Ill* is
understandable when its quirky, wilful, inconsequential musings are set against his much more
austere, authoritative, and classical essay-writing.
He preferred impersonality and logical argument.
But Woolf deliberately modelled her essay-writing
on the Romantic essayists, Hazlitt, Lamb, De
Quincey, Coleridge, who are all involved with *On
Being Ill*. The title echoes Hazlitt—"On Going a
Journey," "On the Fear of Death." (It's a joke, too,
about how often that kind of title gets recycled: in
an earlier essay on "Melodious Meditations," she
teases American essayists for using titles like "Old
Age" and "On Being Ill.")[16] Coleridge's writing on
Shakespeare appears, if only as a faint mouse-
squeak. Charles Lamb's essays and letters, always
great favourites, are in her mind just at this time:
she writes a letter on September 18th, 1925, to her
friend Janet Case, praising Lamb's dashing and
brilliant style, and she quotes one of his letters in the
essay. De Quincey, whom she cites as one of the few

writers on illness, will be her next subject for a
major essay ("Impassioned Prose"), and her first
lavishly cumulative sentence is highly De Quincean
(as are her fantasies about cloud-scapes and her
insistence on our need for solitude). Like these
Romantic essayists, she allows herself deviations
and divagations, though she is more guarded about
herself than they are, more anxious to conceal her
personal experience. But, like them, she uses an intimate, inconsequential speaking voice which makes
the essay read like a form of conversation. Her fan-
tasy, in *On Being Ill*, of a secular, literary after-life
consisting of gossip, conversation, and play-acting,
is enacted in the tone of the essay itself. "I am very
glad you liked my article—" she wrote to a friend
about the essay in February 1926. "I was afraid
that, writing in bed, and forced to write quickly by
the inexorable Tom Eliot I had used too many
words."[17] "Writing in bed" has produced an idio-
syncratic, prolix, recumbent literature—the opposite
of "inexorable"—at once romantic and modern, with
a point of view derived from gazing up at the clouds
and looking sideways on to the world. Illness and
writing are netted together from the very start of
the essay.

Why has illness not been as popular a subject for literature as love, she asks? Why has the "daily drama of the body" not been recognised? Why does literature always insist on separating the mind, or the soul, from the body? Perhaps because the public would never accept illness as a subject for fiction; perhaps because illness requires a new language— "more primitive, more sensual, more obscene." (In the manuscript of the essay, she had "brutal" for "primitive.") But illness is almost impossible to communicate. The invalid's demand for sympathy can never be met. People at once start complaining about their own condition. And, apart from a few (female) eccentrics and misfits (colourfully and rapidly invoked), the world can't afford regular sympathy: it would take up the whole working day. Besides, illness really prefers solitude. "Here we go alone, and like it better so." The ill have dropped out of the army of workers and become deserters. This gives them time to do things normal people can't do, like looking at the clouds or the flowers. And what they find comforting about clouds and flowers is not their sympathy, but their indifference. The ill, unlike the "army of the upright," recognise Nature's indifference; they know Nature is going to win in the end, when ice will bury the world. What consolation is there for that thought? Organised religion? The idea of Heaven? An alternative, secular idea of Heaven, as invented by the poets? And poets (she jumps lightly on) are what we need when ill, not prose writers. "In illness words seem to possess a mystic quality." We are attracted to intense lines and phrases, to the incomprehensible, to the texture of sounds. We make rash readings without critical intermediaries, for instance, of Shakespeare. And if we have enough of him, we can read some trash like Augustus Hare's life of two nineteenth-century aristocratic ladies, which gives us a rush of scenes and stories.

This loose improvisation is netted together by a complex pattern of images, drawing on water, air, earth, and fire, desert wastes and mountain peaks, deep forests and vast seas, clouds, birds, leaves and flowers, as though through illness a whole alternative universe is created. Intensely physical, the writing insists on the body, like a pane of glass, as the transmitter of all experience. The body is monster and hero, animal and mystic, above all actor, in an essay so much about play-acting and scene-making. (Her "cinema" of cloud-scapes, playing "perpetually to an empty house," anticipates a fascinated essay on "The Cinema," published a few months later.)

As the images cohere, a satire on conformity begins to make itself felt. The ill are the deserters, the refuseniks. They won't accept the "co-operative" conventions. They blurt things out. They turn sympathisers away. They won't go to work. They lie down. They waste time. They fantasise. They don't go to Church or believe in Heaven. They refuse to read responsibly or to make sense of what they read. They are attracted to nonsense, sensation, and rashness.[18] On the other side of the glass is "the army of the upright," harnessing energy, driving motor cars, going to work and to church, communicating and civilising. Her prototypes for these good citizens, snatched rather wildly from the newspapers she happens to be reading at the time, are the Bishop of Lichfield, and Samuel Insull, who, before his collapse and disgrace in the Depression years, was co-founder, with Edison, of the General Electric Company, head of the Chicago empire of utility and transportation companies, and the bringer of electrification to "the cities of the Middle West": a wonderful embodiment of productive energy.

Reading in bed, reading when ill—like "writing in bed"—is, it's suggested, a form of deviancy. The theme of rash reading, making one's own "notes in the margin," seems also to allow for rash writing, writing with the apparent wilful inconsequentiality and inconclusiveness of this essay. Since it is as much about reading and writing as it is about illness, this is a very literary essay, full of quotations and allusions. But these are not just decorative tributes to the Romantic essayists, or to Shakespeare. Like her argument, her quotations are not as random as they look. She quotes from Milton's *Comus* ("and oft at eve/Visits the herds along the twilight meadows") part of the description of the goddess Sabrina (just before the invocation that haunts Rachel, in *The Voyage Out*, as she is falling ill), who is implored to help the imprisoned Lady. She quotes from Shelley's *Prometheus Unbound* Asia's recounting of her dream of clouds "wandering in thick flocks along the mountains," as a voice ("low, sweet, faint sounds, like the farewell of ghosts") calls "O follow, follow, follow me." She quotes from an agonised letter of Lamb's, wanting to kill the snake of time, and speaking of his loneliness, desolation, and inertia: "The mind preys on itself...I pity you for

overwork; but I assure you, no work is worse."
She quotes from Rimbaud's poem "O saisons o
châteaux" which made its way into his *Une Saison en
Enfer*, as one of his examples of "verbal hallucinations." It ends with the phrase "l'heure du trépas,"
"the hour of death." She alludes to Shakespeare's
tragedies, especially *Hamlet*. (I read *Hamlet* last
night, she wrote to Vita on 23 September, three
weeks after agreeing to write *On Being Ill*.)[19] *Hamlet*
is in the essay from the beginning, in her reference to
the "undiscovered countries" of illness, and in the
phrase "shuffled off" (used of sympathy). "To be or
not to be" is lurking in the margins. *Antony and
Cleopatra* is there too, in her passage on the shape-
shifting of the clouds, echoing Antony's speech to
Eros about how the clouds unselve themselves, as
he is about to do: "That which is now a horse, even
with a thought/The rack dislimns, and makes it
indistinct/As water is in water."

All these literary echoes point the same way.
Comus, *Prometheus Unbound*, Lamb's letter, Rimbaud,
all have to do with pleas or longing for escape,
struggles with a hell of human anguish and depression. The main Shakespearean allusions are both
about suicide: Hamlet is contemplating it, Antony is

about to commit it. Would Christian faith, she asks
suddenly, give its believers enough conviction "to
leap straight into Heaven off Beachy Head?" (a
well-known suicide spot). Under its playful surface,
there is a muffled, anguished debate going on about
whether illness can take one so far out to sea, so
high up the mountain peak (like Septimus in *Mrs.
Dalloway*), so apart from "normality," that suicide
might seem the only escape.

The last section of the essay (cut from *The
Forum*'s version) seems, at first sight, a peculiar
coda. Why are we being treated to a potted version
of a minor nineteenth-century historian's life of two
unknown aristocratic ladies, jumbled comically
together in the manner Woolf favours for her essays
on "eccentrics" and "obscure lives"? Like so many of
her essays on women ("Geraldine and Jane," "Miss
Ormerod," "Mary Wollstonecraft," *A Room of One's
Own*), this tells the story of a gifted woman suppressed and imprisoned by her circumstances. (And,
for all its scatty, glancing manner, it reproduces
in accurate detail Hare's account of the lives of
Countess Canning and Lady Waterford.) Yet it still
seems a rather random example of desultory reading, until we get to the last image, of the widowed

Lady Waterford, who "crushed together" the plush curtain "in her agony" as she watches her husband's body being taken to his grave.[20] This makes a startling echo of the sick person who, earlier in the essay, has to take his pain in one hand and "a lump of pure sound" in the other and "crush them together" to produce a "brand new word."

"Crushing together" is an action produced by agony. And, both for the invalid mastering illness through language, and the "great lady" mastering her grief, it is an image of fierce courage. "To look these things squarely in the face would need the courage of a lion tamer." ("Of ten thousand lion tamers,—for these lions are within us not without.") Virginia Woolf does not write explicitly about herself; as in almost all her essays, she does not say "I" ("tyrannical 'I'"), but "we," "one," "us." Yet the essay is a demonstration of her heroic powers of endurance and courage, her lack of self-pity, and the use she made of her physical and mental suffering, every bit as productive as Mr. Insull: how she put them to work, and transformed them into a new kind of writing.

HERMIONE LEE
APRIL 15, 2002

NOTES

1. For a fuller account of this, see my *Virginia Woolf*, Chatto & Windus, 1996, Ch. 10. N.B. also Thomas Caramagno, *The Flight of the Mind: Virginia Woolf's Art and Manic-Depressive Illness*, University of California Press, 1992, 13, on how "anxiety-depression can mimic many diseases or disorders," and quoting Emil Kraepelin on the frequency of headaches in manic-depressive patients.

2. *The Diary of Virginia Woolf*, ed. Anne Olivier Bell, assisted by Andrew McNeillie, The Hogarth Press, 1980 [*Diary*], 16 February 1930, III, 287.

3. *Diary*, 5 September 1925, III, 38.

4. *Diary*, 5 September 1925, III, 38; Letter to Vita Sackville-West [VSW], 7 September 1925, *The Letters of Virginia Woolf*, ed. Nigel Nicolson, assist. ed. Joanne Trautmann, The Hogarth Press, 1977 [*Letters*], III, 205; *Diary*, 14 September 1925, III, 40; Letter to Roger Fry, 16 September 1925, *Letters*, III, 208; Letter to VSW, 13 October 1925, *Letters*, III, 217; Letter to VSW, 26? October 1925, *Letters*, III, 218; Letter to VSW, 16 November 1925, *Letters*, III, 221; *Diary*, 27 November 1925, III, 46.

5. *Diary*, 27 November 1925, III, 47.

6. *Diary*, 14 September 1925, III, 41.

7. Letter to T. S. Eliot, 3 [should be 8] September 1925, *Letters*, III, 203.

8. Letter to T. S. Eliot, 13 November 1925, *Letters*, III, 220.

9. *Diary*, 7 December 1925, III, 49.

10. T. S. Eliot, "The Idea of a Literary Review," Preface, *New Criterion*, IV (January 1925-1926), Faber & Gwyer.

11. *The Forum*, Vol. LXXV, No. 4, April 1926.

12. It made three other significant alterations. The list of diseases that

ought to be a fit subject for literature included "Appendicitis and Cancer." The need to have "the courage of a lion tamer" to look illness in the face went on: "of ten thousand lion tamers,—for these lions are within us not without." And the names of the alternative lives we might live as "William or Alice" became (linking it with an earlier passage), "Mrs. Jones or Mr. Smith."

13. *Diary*, 2 September 1930, III, 315.

14. VW to "Anon," 10 December 1930, *Letters*, IV, 260. See John H. Willis, Jr., *Leonard and Virginia Woolf as Publishers: The Hogarth Press*, 1917-41, University Press of Virginia, 1992, 34.

15. See *Virginia Woolf and the Essay*, eds. Beth Carole Rosenberg and Jeanne Dubino, St. Martin's Press, 1997; Juliet Dusinberre, *Virginia Woolf's Renaissance*, Macmillan, 1997.

16. "Melodious Meditations," 1917, *The Essays of Virginia Woolf* [*Essays*], ed. Andrew McNeillie, The Hogarth Press, 1987, Vol. II, 80.

17. Letter to Edward Sackville-West, 6 February 1926, *Letters*, III, 239-240.

18. Cf. "In order to read poetry rightly, one must be in a rash, an extreme, a generous state of mind." "How Should One Read a Book?" given as a lecture on 26 January 1926 (in the same month as the publication of *On Being Ill*). *Essays*, III, 395.

19. Letter to Vita Sackville-West, 23 September 1925, *Letters*, III, 215.

20. Here she improves on her source, which has a "window blind" rather than a plush curtain: "This blind told me of her intense suffering, for there was the clutch of her fingers, as they wrinkled the surface in her anguish. There was writing in the folds caused by her squeeze that told more than words could of the heart's despair." Augustus Hare, *The Story of Two Noble Lives. Being Memorials of Charlotte, Countess Canning, and Louisa, Marchioness of Waterford*, London, George Allen, 1893, Vol. III, 23-24.

ON BEING ILL

Considering how common illness is, how tremendous the spiritual change that it brings, how astonishing, when the lights of health go down, the undiscovered countries that are then disclosed, what wastes and deserts of the soul a slight attack of influenza brings to view, what precipices and lawns sprinkled with bright flowers a little rise of temperature reveals, what ancient and obdurate oaks are uprooted in us by the act of sickness, how we go down into the pit of death and feel the waters of annihilation close above our heads and wake thinking to find ourselves in the presence of the angels and the harpers when we have a tooth out and come to the surface in the dentist's arm-chair and confuse his "Rinse the mouth—rinse the mouth" with the greeting of the Deity stooping from the floor of Heaven to welcome us—when we think of this, as we are so frequently forced to think of it, it becomes strange indeed that illness has not taken its place with love and battle and

jealousy among the prime themes of literature.
Novels, one would have thought, would have
been devoted to influenza; epic poems to typhoid; odes to pneumonia; lyrics to toothache.
But no; with a few exceptions—De Quincey
attempted something of the sort in *The Opium
Eater*; there must be a volume or two about
disease scattered through the pages of
Proust—literature does its best to maintain
that its concern is with the mind; that the body
is a sheet of plain glass through which the soul
looks straight and clear, and, save for one
or two passions such as desire and greed, is
null, and negligible and non-existent. On the
contrary, the very opposite is true. All day, all
night the body intervenes; blunts or sharpens,
colours or discolours, turns to wax in the
warmth of June, hardens to tallow in the murk
of February. The creature within can only gaze
through the pane—smudged or rosy; it cannot
separate off from the body like the sheath of a
knife or the pod of a pea for a single instant; it

must go through the whole unending procession of changes, heat and cold, comfort and discomfort, hunger and satisfaction, health and illness, until there comes the inevitable catastrophe; the body smashes itself to smithereens, and the soul (it is said) escapes. But of all this daily drama of the body there is no record. People write always of the doings of the mind; the thoughts that come to it; its noble plans; how the mind has civilised the universe. They show it ignoring the body in the philosopher's turret; or kicking the body, like an old leather football, across leagues of snow and desert in the pursuit of conquest or discovery. Those great wars which the body wages with the mind a slave to it, in the solitude of the bedroom against the assault of fever or the oncome of melancholia, are neglected. Nor is the reason far to seek. To look these things squarely in the face would need the courage of a lion tamer; a robust philosophy; a reason rooted in the bowels of the earth.

Short of these, this monster, the body, this miracle, its pain, will soon make us taper into mysticism, or rise, with rapid beats of the wings, into the raptures of transcendentalism. The public would say that a novel devoted to influenza lacked plot; they would complain that there was no love in it—wrongly however, for illness often takes on the disguise of love, and plays the same odd tricks. It invests certain faces with divinity, sets us to wait, hour after hour, with pricked ears for the creaking of a stair, and wreathes the faces of the absent (plain enough in health, Heaven knows) with a new significance, while the mind concocts a thousand legends and romances about them for which it has neither time nor taste in health. Finally, to hinder the description of illness in literature, there is the poverty of the language. English, which can express the thoughts of Hamlet and the tragedy of Lear, has no words for the shiver and the headache. It has all grown one way. The merest schoolgirl, when

she falls in love, has Shakespeare or Keats to
speak her mind for her; but let a sufferer try to
describe a pain in his head to a doctor and language at once runs dry. There is nothing ready
made for him. He is forced to coin words himself, and, taking his pain in one hand, and a
lump of pure sound in the other (as perhaps
the people of Babel did in the beginning), so to
crush them together that a brand new word in
the end drops out. Probably it will be something laughable. For who of English birth can
take liberties with the language? To us it is a
sacred thing and therefore doomed to die,
unless the Americans, whose genius is so much
happier in the making of new words than in the
disposition of the old, will come to our help
and set the springs aflow. Yet it is not only a
new language that we need, more primitive,
more sensual, more obscene, but a new hier-
archy of the passions; love must be deposed in
favour of a temperature of 104; jealousy give
place to the pangs of sciatica; sleeplessness play

the part of villain, and the hero become a white
liquid with a sweet taste—that mighty Prince
with the moths' eyes and the feathered feet, one
of whose names is Chloral.

But to return to the invalid. "I am in bed
with influenza"—but what does that convey
of the great experience; how the world has
changed its shape; the tools of business grown
remote; the sounds of festival become romantic
like a merry-go-round heard across far fields;
and friends have changed, some putting on
a strange beauty, others deformed to the
squatness of toads, while the whole landscape
of life lies remote and fair, like the shore seen
from a ship far out at sea, and he is now exalted on a peak and needs no help from man or
God, and now grovels supine on the floor glad
of a kick from a housemaid—the experience
cannot be imparted and, as is always the way
with these dumb things, his own suffering
serves but to wake memories in his friends'
minds of *their* influenzas, *their* aches and pains

which went unwept last February, and now cry
aloud, desperately, clamorously, for the divine
relief of sympathy.

But sympathy we cannot have. Wisest Fate
says no. If her children, weighted as they
already are with sorrow, were to take on them
that burden too, adding in imagination other
pains to their own, buildings would cease to
rise; roads would peter out into grassy tracks;
there would be an end of music and of paint-
ing; one great sigh alone would rise to Heaven,
and the only attitudes for men and women
would be those of horror and despair. As it
is, there is always some little distraction—an
organ grinder at the corner of the hospital, a
shop with book or trinket to decoy one past
the prison or the workhouse, some absurdity
of cat or dog to prevent one from turning
the old beggar's hieroglyphic of misery into
volumes of sordid suffering; and thus the vast
effort of sympathy which those barracks
of pain and discipline, those dried symbols of

sorrow, ask us to exert on their behalf, is uneasily shuffled off for another time. Sympathy nowadays is dispensed chiefly by the laggards and failures, women for the most part (in whom the obsolete exists so strangely side by side with anarchy and newness), who, having dropped out of the race, have time to spend upon fantastic and unprofitable excursions; C. L. for example, who, sitting by the stale sickroom fire, builds up, with touches at once sober and imaginative, the nursery fender, the loaf, the lamp, barrel organs in the street, and all the simple old wives' tales of pinafores and escapades; A. R., the rash, the magnanimous, who, if you fancied a giant tortoise to solace you or theorbo to cheer you, would ransack the markets of London and procure them somehow, wrapped in paper, before the end of the day; the frivolous K. T., who, dressed in silks and feathers, powdered and painted (which takes time too) as if for a banquet of Kings and Queens, spends her whole brightness in the

gloom of the sick room, and makes the medicine bottles ring and the flames shoot up with
her gossip and her mimicry. But such follies
have had their day; civilisation points to a
different goal; and then what place will there
be for the tortoise and the theorbo?

There is, let us confess it (and illness is the
great confessional), a childish outspokenness in
illness; things are said, truths blurted out,
which the cautious respectability of health con-
ceals. About sympathy for example—we can do
without it. That illusion of a world so shaped
that it echoes every groan, of human beings
so tied together by common needs and fears
that a twitch at one wrist jerks another, where
however strange your experience other people
have had it too, where however far you travel
in your own mind someone has been there
before you—is all an illusion. We do not know
our own souls, let alone the souls of others.
Human beings do not go hand in hand the
whole stretch of the way. There is a virgin

forest in each; a snowfield where even the print of birds' feet is unknown. Here we go alone, and like it better so. Always to have sympathy, always to be accompanied, always to be understood would be intolerable. But in health the genial pretense must be kept up and the effort renewed—to communicate, to civilise, to share, to cultivate the desert, educate the native, to work together by day and by night to sport. In illness this make-believe ceases. Directly the bed is called for, or, sunk deep among pillows in one chair, we raise our feet even an inch above the ground on another, we cease to be soldiers in the army of the upright; we become deserters. They march to battle. We float with the sticks on the stream; helter-skelter with the dead leaves on the lawn, irresponsible and disinterested and able, perhaps for the first time for years, to look round, to look up—to look, for example, at the sky.

The first impression of that extraordinary spectacle is strangely overcoming. Ordinarily

to look at the sky for any length of time
is impossible. Pedestrians would be impeded
and disconcerted by a public sky-gazer. What
snatches we get of it are mutilated by chimneys
and churches, serve as a background for man,
signify wet weather or fine, daub windows
gold, and, filling in the branches, complete the
pathos of dishevelled autumnal plane trees in
autumnal squares. Now, lying recumbent, star-
ing straight up, the sky is discovered to be
something so different from this that really it
is a little shocking. This then has been going
on all the time without our knowing it!—this
incessant making up of shapes and casting
them down, this buffeting of clouds together,
and drawing vast trains of ships and waggons
from North to South, this incessant ringing
up and down of curtains of light and shade,
this interminable experiment with gold shafts
and blue shadows, with veiling the sun and
unveiling it, with making rock ramparts and
wafting them away—this endless activity, with

the waste of Heaven knows how many million
horse power of energy, has been left to work its
will year in year out. The fact seems to call for
comment and indeed for censure. Ought not
some one to write to *The Times*? Use should be
made of it. One should not let this gigantic
cinema play perpetually to an empty house.
But watch a little longer and another emotion
drowns the stirrings of civic ardour. Divinely
beautiful it is also divinely heartless. Immeasur-
able resources are used for some purpose
which has nothing to do with human pleasure
or human profit. If we were all laid prone, stiff,
still the sky would be experimenting with its
blues and its golds. Perhaps then, if we look
down at something very small and close and
familiar, we shall find sympathy. Let us exam-
ine the rose. We have seen it so often flowering
in bowls, connected it so often with beauty in
its prime, that we have forgotten how it stands,
still and steady, throughout an entire afternoon in the earth. It preserves a demeanour

of perfect dignity and self-possession. The
suffusion of its petals is of inimitable rightness.
Now perhaps one deliberately falls; now all the
flowers, the voluptuous purple, the creamy, in
whose waxen flesh the spoon has left a swirl of
cherry juice; gladioli; dahlias; lilies, sacerdotal,
ecclesiastical; flowers with prim cardboard col-
lars tinged apricot and amber, all gently incline
their heads to the breeze—all, with the excep-
tion of the heavy sunflower, who proudly
acknowledges the sun at midday and perhaps
at midnight rebuffs the moon. There they
stand; and it is of these, the stillest, the most
self-sufficient of all things that human beings
have made companions; these that symbolise
their passions, decorate their festivals, and lie
(as if *they* knew sorrow) upon the pillows of
the dead. Wonderful to relate, poets have
found religion in nature; people live in the
country to learn virtue from plants. It is in
their indifference that they are comforting.
That snowfield of the mind, where man has not

trodden, is visited by the cloud, kissed by the falling petal, as, in another sphere, it is the great artists, the Miltons and the Popes, who console not by their thought of us but by their forgetfulness.

Meanwhile, with the heroism of the ant or the bee, however indifferent the sky or disdainful the flowers, the army of the upright marches to battle. Mrs. Jones catches her train. Mr. Smith mends his motor. The cows are driven home to be milked. Men thatch the roof. The dogs bark. The rooks, rising in a net, fall in a net upon the elm trees. The wave of life flings itself out indefatigably. It is only the recumbent who know what, after all, Nature is at no pains to conceal—that she in the end will conquer; heat will leave the world; stiff with frost we shall cease to drag ourselves about the fields; ice will lie thick upon factory and engine; the sun will go out. Even so, when the whole earth is sheeted and slippery, some undulation, some irregularity of surface will mark the boundary of an ancient garden, and there, thrusting its head up undaunted in the starlight, the rose will flower, the crocus will burn. But with the hook of life still in us still we must wriggle. We cannot stiffen peaceably into glassy mounds. Even the recumbent spring up at the mere imagination of frost about the toes and stretch out to avail themselves of the universal hope—Heaven, Immortality. Surely, since men have been wishing all these ages, they will have wished something into existence; there will be some green isle for the mind to rest on even if the foot cannot plant itself there. The co-operative imagination of mankind must have drawn some firm outline. But no. One opens the *Morning Post* and reads the Bishop of Lichfield on Heaven. One watches the church-goers file into those gallant temples where, on the bleakest day, in the wettest fields, lamps will be burning, bells will be ringing, and however the autumn leaves may shuffle and the winds sigh

outside, hopes and desires will be changed to
beliefs and certainties within. Do they look
serene? Are their eyes filled with the light of
their supreme conviction? Would one of them
dare leap straight into Heaven off Beachy
Head? None but a simpleton would ask such
questions; the little company of believers lags
and drags and strays. The mother is worn; the
father tired. As for imagining Heaven, they
have no time. Heaven-making must be left to
the imagination of the poets. Without their
help we can but trifle—imagine Pepys in
Heaven, adumbrate little interviews with cele-
brated people on tufts of thyme, soon fall into
gossip about such of our friends as have stayed
in Hell, or, worse still, revert again to earth
and choose, since there is no harm in choosing,
to live over and over, now as man, now as
woman, as sea-captain, or court lady, as
Emperor or farmer's wife, in splendid cities
and on remote moors, at the time of Pericles or
Arthur, Charlemagne, or George the Fourth—

to live and live till we have lived out those embryo lives which attend about us in early youth until "I" suppressed them. But "I" shall not, if wishing can alter it, usurp Heaven too, and condemn us, who have played our parts here as William or Alice to remain William or Alice for ever. Left to ourselves we speculate thus carnally. We need the poets to imagine for us. The duty of Heaven-making should be attached to the office of the Poet Laureate.

Indeed it is to the poets that we turn. Illness makes us disinclined for the long campaigns that prose exacts. We cannot command all our faculties and keep our reason and our judgment and our memory at attention while chapter swings on top of chapter, and, as one settles into place, we must be on the watch for the coming of the next, until the whole structure—arches, towers, and battlements— stands firm on its foundations. *The Decline and Fall of the Roman Empire* is not the book for influenza, nor *The Golden Bowl* nor *Madame*

Bovary. On the other hand, with responsibility shelved and reason in the abeyance—for who is going to exact criticism from an invalid or sound sense from the bed-ridden?—other tastes assert themselves; sudden, fitful, intense. We rifle the poets of their flowers. We break off a line or two and let them open in the depths of the mind:

> *and oft at eve*
> *Visits the herds along the twilight meadows*
>
> *wandering in thick flocks along the mountains*
> *Shepherded by the slow unwilling wind.*

Or there is a whole three volume novel to be mused over in a verse of Hardy's or a sentence of La Bruyère. We dip in Lamb's Letters— some prose writers are to be read as poets— and find "I am a sanguinary murderer of time, and would kill him inchmeal just now. But the snake is vital." and who shall explain the delight? or open Rimbaud and read

O saisons o châteaux
Quelle âme est sans défauts?

and who shall rationalise the charm? In illness
words seem to possess a mystic quality. We
grasp what is beyond their surface meaning,
gather instinctively this, that, and the other—a
sound, a colour, here a stress, there a pause—
which the poet, knowing words to be meagre in
comparison with ideas, has strewn about his
page to evoke, when collected, a state of mind
which neither words can express nor the reason
explain. Incomprehensibility has an enormous
power over us in illness, more legitimately perhaps than the upright will allow. In health
meaning has encroached upon sound. Our
intelligence domineers over our senses. But in
illness, with the police off duty, we creep
beneath some obscure poem by Mallarmé
or Donne, some phrase in Latin or Greek,
and the words give out their scent and distil
their flavour, and then, if at last we grasp the

meaning, it is all the richer for having come to us sensually first, by way of the palate and the nostrils, like some queer odour. Foreigners, to whom the tongue is strange, have us at a disadvantage. The Chinese must know the sound of *Antony and Cleopatra* better than we do.

Rashness is one of the properties of illness—outlaws that we are—and it is rashness that we need in reading Shakespeare. It is not that we should doze in reading him, but that, fully conscious and aware, his fame intimidates and bores, and all the views of all the critics dull in us that thunder clap of conviction which, if an illusion, is still so helpful an illusion, so prodigious a pleasure, so keen a stimulus in reading the great. Shakespeare is getting flyblown; a paternal government might well forbid writing about him, as they put his monument at Stratford beyond the reach of scribbling fingers. With all this buzz of criticism about, one may hazard one's conjectures privately, make one's notes in the margin; but, knowing that someone has said it before, or said it better, the zest is gone. Illness, in its kingly sublimity, sweeps all that aside and leaves nothing but Shakespeare and oneself. What with his overweening power and our overweening arrogance, the barriers go down, the knots run smooth, the brain rings and resounds with *Lear* or *Macbeth*, and even Coleridge himself squeaks like a distant mouse.

But enough of Shakespeare—let us turn to Augustus Hare. There are people who say that even illness does not warrant these transitions; that the author of *The Story of Two Noble Lives* is not the peer of Boswell; and if we assert that short of the best in literature we like the worst—it is mediocrity that is hateful—will have none of that either. So be it. The law is on the side of the normal. But for those who suffer a slight rise of temperature the names of Hare and Waterford and Canning ray out as beams of benignant lustre. Not, it is true, for

the first hundred pages or so. There, as so
often in these fat volumes, we flounder and
threaten to sink in a plethora of aunts and
uncles. We have to remind ourselves that there
is such a thing as atmosphere; that the masters
themselves often keep us waiting intolerably
while they prepare our minds for whatever it
may be—the surprise, or the lack of surprise.
So Hare, too, takes his time; the charm steals
upon us imperceptibly; by degrees we become
almost one of the family, yet not quite, for our
sense of the oddity of it all remains, and share
the family dismay when Lord Stuart leaves the
room—there was a ball going forward—and
is next heard of in Iceland. Parties, he said,
bored him—such were English aristocrats
before marriage with intellect had adulterated
the fine singularity of their minds. Parties bore
them; they are off to Iceland. Then Beckford's
mania for castle building attacked him; he
must lift a French *château* across the Channel,
and erect pinnacles and towers to use as

servants' bedrooms at vast expense, upon the
borders of a crumbling cliff, too, so that the
housemaids saw their brooms swimming down
the Solent, and Lady Stuart was much dis-
tressed, but made the best of it and began,
like the high-born lady that she was, planting
evergreens in the face of ruin. Meanwhile
the daughters, Charlotte and Louisa, grew up
in their incomparable loveliness, with pencils
in their hands, for ever sketching, dancing,
flirting, in a cloud of gauze. They are not very
distinct it is true. For life then was not the life
of Charlotte and Louisa. It was the life of
families, of groups. It was a web, a net, spread-
ing wide and enmeshing every sort of cousin,
dependant, and old retainer. Aunts—Aunt
Caledon, Aunt Mexborough—grandmothers—
Granny Stuart, Granny Hardwicke—cluster
in chorus, and rejoice and sorrow and eat
Christmas dinner together, and grow very old
and remain very upright, and sit in hooded
chairs cutting flowers it seems out of coloured

paper. Charlotte married Canning and went to
India; Louisa married Lord Waterford and
went to Ireland. Then letters begin to cross
vast spaces in slow sailing ships and communi-
cation becomes still more protracted and
verbose, and there seems no end to the space
and the leisure of those early Victorian days,
and faiths are lost and the life of Hedley
Vicars revives them; aunts catch cold but
recover; cousins marry; there are the Irish
famine and the Indian Mutiny, and both sisters
remain to their great, but silent, grief without
children to come after them. Louisa, dumped
down in Ireland with Lord Waterford at the
hunt all day, was often very lonely; but she
stuck to her post, visited the poor, spoke
words of comfort ("I am sorry indeed to hear
of Anthony Thompson's loss of mind, or
rather of memory; if, however, he can under-
stand sufficiently to trust solely in our Saviour,
he has enough") and sketched and sketched.
Thousands of notebooks were filled with pen

and ink drawings of an evening, and then the
carpenter stretched sheets for her and she
designed frescoes for schoolrooms, had live
sheep into her bedroom, draped gamekeepers
in blankets, painted Holy Families in abun-
dance, until the great Watts exclaimed that
here was Titian's peer and Raphael's master!
At that Lady Waterford laughed (she had a
generous, benignant sense of humour); and
said that she was nothing but a sketcher; had
scarcely had a lesson in her life—witness her
angel's wings scandalously unfinished. More-
over, there was her father's house forever
falling into the sea; she must shore it up; must
entertain her friends; must fill her days with all
sorts of charities, till her Lord came home
from hunting, and then, at midnight often, she
would sketch him with his knightly face half
hidden in a bowl of soup, sitting with her
sketch-book under a lamp beside him. Off he
would ride again, stately as a crusader, to hunt
the fox, and she would wave to him and think

each time, what if this should be the last? And
so it was, that winter's morning; his horse
stumbled; he was killed. She knew it before
they told her, and never could Sir John Leslie
forget, when he ran downstairs on the day of
the burial, the beauty of the great lady standing to see the hearse depart, nor, when he came
back, how the curtain, heavy, mid-Victorian,
plush perhaps, was all crushed together where
she had grasped it in her agony.

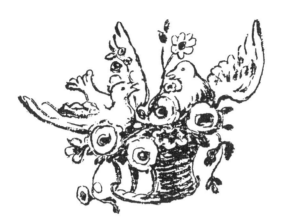

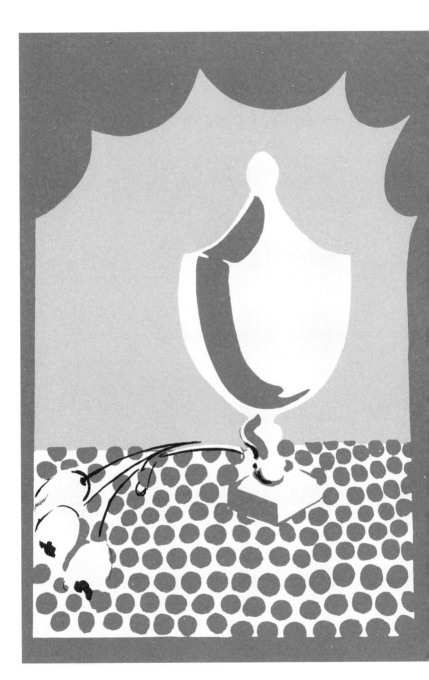

NOTES FROM SICK ROOMS

INTRODUCTION

"WE THINK BACK through our mothers, if we are women," Virginia Woolf wrote in *A Room of One's Own*. But who was the mother Woolf herself thought "back through"? Bringing together Woolf's *On Being Ill* and Julia Stephen's *Notes from Sick Rooms* in a single volume gives us an extraordinary opportunity to hear a kind of dialogue between Woolf and her mother, who died when she was just thirteen. Stephen's detailed manual of instruction—for those who find themselves caring for a sick person—foreshadows the wit and sharp observation that is so characteristic of her famous daughter's style. *Notes from Sick Rooms* also demonstrates an attentiveness to the ways that illness influences our perception, which Woolf discusses throughout *On Being Ill*. In *On Being Ill*, Woolf laments that literature has largely neglected the "daily drama of the body" during illness. *Notes from Sick Rooms* is filled with commentary on that very drama, played out every hour in the presence of the nurse caring for that body.

In "A Sketch of the Past," a memoir Woolf began in 1939, she describes her mother at "the very centre of that great Cathedral space which is childhood."[1] This centrality is recalled by the character of Mrs. Ramsay in Woolf's 1927 novel *To the Lighthouse*, the first part of which Woolf was writing when she composed *On Being Ill*. Like Julia Stephen, Mrs. Ramsay presides over a household of eight children, an irascible husband, and numerous servants and guests. Like Julia, Mrs. Ramsay adds to her domestic demands a wide circle of charitable visits to the poor and sick, a pattern that was set early in Woolf's mother's life.

Julia was born in India in 1846, the third daughter of John Jackson, a medical doctor, and Maria Pattle. Returning with her mother to England in 1848, Julia grew up among the painters and poets, novelists and philosophers who frequented both her uncle Henry Thoby Prinsep's Little Holland House, and her aunt Julia Margaret Cameron's house, Freshwater, on the Isle of Wight. A pioneering photographer, Julia Margaret Cameron created images of her niece Julia that contributed to her reputation as an extraordinary beauty.[2] Maria Pattle suffered from rheumatism, and after the marriages of her two elder daughters, it was sixteen-year-old Julia who became her mother's nurse and companion on trips seeking a cure for her illness. In Venice, on one such excursion, Julia met Herbert Duckworth, a young barrister whom she married in 1867 at the age of twenty-one. That same year Woolf's father, Leslie Stephen, married Minny, the younger daughter of the novelist William Make-peace Thackeray.

Julia's idyllic marriage to Herbert Duckworth ended when she was twenty-four and pregnant with her third child. Herbert reached to pick a fig from a tree; an abscess ruptured, and he quickly died. Six weeks later, Gerald was born, a circumstance that prevented Julia from revealing her despair. Herbert's sudden death left her "deadened," but she had to "keep up" for the sake of her baby. "If it had been possible for me to be myself," she wrote to Leslie Stephen, "it would have been better for me individually...I could never be alone which sometimes was such torture."[3] In the aftermath of Herbert's death, she lost her religious faith, and found sympathetic support in reading Leslie Stephen's influential essays on agnosticism. Stephen had resigned his position at Cambridge University in 1862 because he could not reconcile his religious doubts with the University's requirement that he become ordained in the Anglican Church. By 1866 he was writing regularly on religious matters in *Fraser's Magazine*.

On the evening of November 27th, 1875, Julia called on Minny and Leslie Stephen. She was close friends with Minny's sister Anny, a writer whose stories and essays she often helped to edit. The next day, on Leslie's forty-third birthday, Minny died of a seizure, pregnant with her second child. During the next two years, Julia and Leslie became friends, sharing their agnosticism and the bereavement for their spouses. From the beginning of their friendship, Julia made it clear that she would never marry again. Over time, however, Julia fell in love with Leslie, and in 1878 she agreed to become his wife. The wedding date was set for March 7th, but "we have had to put it off till (probably) the 26th. [Julia] was suddenly summoned to the deathbed of an uncle, who had been almost a father to her," wrote Leslie to his close friend Charles Eliot Norton, the American intellectual and professor of art history at Harvard. This was not unusual for Julia, Leslie explains in his letter to Norton: "she has been so accustomed to look after sick people that I am

always expecting some of her cousins or aunts or
uncles to get into trouble & send for her at a
moment's notice....She has at the moment 3 sets of
relatives sick: 1 niece with pleurisy; 2 nieces & a
nephew with scarlet fever & measles; 1 aunt in need
of a surgical operation & all calling for help!"[4] In
Leslie's opinion, Julia felt less strongly about her
father than about her mother because Dr. Jackson
"had never had a day's illness in his life."[5]

   Julia epitomized the Victorian middle-class fem-
inine ideal of "the angel in the house." In her essay
"Professions for Women," Woolf said that before
she could write what she wanted she had to kill this
phantom of Victorian womanhood that whispered in
her ear how she must always care for those in need
and be sympathetic to men. The phrase "angel in the
house" is the title of a long sequence of poems by the
Victorian poet Coventry Patmore. Julia Stephen
owned a copy of *The Angel in the House* inscribed to
her "with the kind regard of" the author, who was a
friend of her mother's. The ideology that strictly
divided the separate spheres of women's and men's
roles was promoted by many writers of the period,
but Patmore's phrase captured that mixture of self-
lessness and sentiment which characterized the

woman who always put her own needs last, who soothed men's troubled brows, and who was solely responsible for the harmony of the domestic hearth. Caring for the sick was regarded as a natural quality of a true Victorian woman.

Virginia Woolf could not remember ever being alone with her mother "except for a moment if one were ill or in some child's crisis."[6] Her sister Vanessa Bell also remarked that "children on the whole love being ill."[7] In a story written for her own children, Julia herself seems to have recognized the truth of her daughters' observations. In "Cat's Meat," Bob and Maggie wonder when they will see their mother because she is so often away from home, "looking after some poor people." Even when home, "she seemed as if she had left part of herself somewhere else." The siblings plan to run away so that "now we shall be the poor, we shall be others, and so she will come and look after us."[8]

In "A Sketch of the Past," Virginia Woolf says that her mother died "without leaving a book, or a picture, or any piece of work," perhaps deeming the writing that Julia in fact did leave too slight for posterity's notice. Ten years after their mother's untimely death at the age of forty-nine, Julia's four

younger children returned to St. Ives, the seaside
town in Cornwall where the family had spent their
summers from 1881 until 1895. On a rainy August
afternoon in 1905, Virginia and her younger
brother, Adrian, took shelter in the fifteenth-
century parish church. An old woman by the door
began to weep when they mentioned their mother's
name: "to have left so deep an impression...,"
Woolf wrote in her diary, "that after eleven years
tears will start at the thought of all the beauty &
charity that are recalled by a name seems to me perhaps the purest tribute which can be paid to the
nobility of a life which did not seek for any other
fortune."[9] In "A Sketch," Woolf recorded a more
tangible tribute to her mother in the form of the
Julia Prinsep Stephen Nursing Association which
still existed in St. Ives in 1940.[10]

From a young age, Julia had observed a skilled
practitioner of what she describes in *Notes from Sick
Rooms* as the "art of being ill": her mother. Maria
Pattle Jackson would typically use three pages of a
four-page letter to her daughter for an intimate
report on the state of her health.[11] By the time
Leslie Stephen married Julia, he described her as "a
kind of sister of mercy" who was always the first to

be called whenever someone in the family died or was ill.[12] Two years after Julia's death, an announcement in *The Nursing Record & Hospital World* sought subscriptions for the Julia Prinsep Stephen Nursing Fund. A "suitable memorial to this lady," it stated on May 1st, 1897, would secure the continuing services of a district nurse in St. Ives, which had no hospital.[13] Sir Leslie Stephen agreed that the fund was "the best memorial of my beloved," and contributed £200.[14]

It is certain that Julia Stephen was familiar with Florence Nightingale's activities in hospitals, and her immensely popular *Notes on Nursing* (which sold 15,000 copies the month it was published). Florence Nightingale claimed that "every woman is a nurse" because she "has, at one time or another of her life, charge of the personal health of somebody, whether child or invalid."[15] Julia Stephen concurred, and recorded her observations and experiences in *Notes from Sick Rooms*, making clear that she claimed no professional status or medical knowledge, but emphasizing that wisdom learned through practice could benefit anyone who had to care for an ill person. The professional training of nurses began to be discussed as early as the 1820s, yet even for

Nightingale, care of the sick remained a vocation rather than a profession: her book embodied knowledge which she believed anyone caring for a sick person should have, but she distinguished that from "medical knowledge, which only a profession can have." The "angel in the house" was *naturally* disposed to caring for others. When "An Appeal Against Female Suffrage" was published in 1889, which argued that giving women the vote would damage their "true dignity and special mission," Virginia Woolf's mother signed it.

In 1880, Julia wrote a response, never published, to the argument put forward by Mrs. Bertha Lathbury in the *Nineteenth Century* that agnostic women would not enter the sick room because they had no religious call to such duty. Julia's response comments on an issue that has been revisited recently in American political discourse: can we expect to find good works without roots in religious faith? The motivation of a nurse is not heavenly reward, wrote Julia: "We are bound to these sufferers by the tie of sisterhood and while life lasts we will help, soothe, and, if we can, love them. Pity has no creed, suffering no limits."[16] She wrote in *Notes from Sick Rooms* that illness "has, or ought to have,

much of the levelling power of death." A sick person is a "case," and all the vagaries of personality,
the irritations of habit, are forgotten in the sick
room where one person is called to care for another.

Julia emphasizes the point of view of the sick
person as paramount in care, distinguishing that
care from medical attention. In *Notes from Sick
Rooms*, she states that distances do not appear the
same to a person confined to bed as they do to those
who are upright. Perceptions of draughts or smells
should not be discounted by the nurse. "Nothing is
small in illness," she writes; when a sick person
finds it difficult to find the right words, the nurse
must be patient for "the mind moves slowly to
expression in illness, and the feeling that the words
are impatiently waited for takes away the power to
utter them." Like Florence Nightingale, Julia
Stephen emphasizes that only the sick person knows
how she feels; therefore, if the arrangement of pillows looks as if it cannot possibly be comfortable,
leave them alone because only the person in the bed
can know they are placed just right. Julia also favors
telling the truth to a sick person to avoid the greater
misery of imagined catastrophes. When circum-

stances demand it, however, the nurse is encouraged to "lie freely."

Woolf demonstrated her own facility in such strategic lying when in 1906 she maintained for a month after his death that her brother Thoby was getting better. In letter after letter to her friend Violet Dickinson, suffering from the same typhoid that killed Thoby, Woolf wrote that "there isn't much change"; that he was "improving"; that he was complaining his nurses wouldn't let him eat mutton. When Violet happened to see a reference to Thoby's death in a newspaper, Woolf wrote on December 18th, "Do you hate me for telling so many lies? You know we had to do it."[17] In her first novel, which she had likely already begun by 1906, Woolf describes a scene that echoes the simple, practical care described in *Notes from Sick Rooms*, while introducing the title character of her later novel, *Mrs. Dalloway*:

> Pale agonies crossed Mrs. Dalloway in waves. When the curtains flapped, grey lights puffed across her. Between the spasms of the storm, Helen made the curtain fast, shook the pillows,

stretched the bed-clothes, and smoothed the hot
nostrils and forehead with cold scent.

"You *are* good!" Clarissa gasped. "Horrid
mess!"

She was trying to apologise for white under-
clothes fallen and scattered on the floor. For one
second she opened a single eye, and saw that the
room was tidy. "That's nice," she gasped. (*The
Voyage Out*)

After reading *Notes from Sick Rooms*, Woolf's
first biographer, Winifred Holtby, saw at once
"clear proof that Virginia inherited the instinct to
write from her mother as well as from her father."
Julia's wonderful passage on crumbs in the sick bed,
a phenomenon that has eluded the powers of scientific explanation, could have been written by Virginia Woolf. "Mrs. Stephen," like her daughter,
"must have had ample opportunity of listening to
philosophers determining the origin of most things,
yet ignoring completely the possible explanation of
crumbs," Holtby observes.[18] This agnostic woman
of the second half of the nineteenth century's gentle
mockery of learned men's inability to account for
the origin of crumbs foreshadows her daughter's

feminist comedy. We can hear echoes of Julia's humor in a passage from *A Room of One's Own*: "How much thinking those old gentlemen used to save one! How the borders of ignorance shrank back at their approach! Cats do not go to heaven! Women cannot write the plays of Shakespeare!"

IN A SHORT memoir written after her sister Virginia's death, Vanessa Bell recalled a time when all four Stephen children had whooping cough and had to be nursed together: "The rest of us quickly recovered, but it seemed to me that Virginia was different. She...had actually entered into some new layer of consciousness rather abruptly, and was suddenly aware of all sorts of questions and possibilities hitherto closed to her." When Woolf wrote *On Being Ill*, she was in the most intense period of her love affair with Vita Sackville-West, who, she confided to her diary, "lavishes on me the maternal protection which, for some reason, is what I have always most wished from everyone."[19] In *Notes from Sick Rooms*, her own often absent mother refers to the "many terrors which haunt the helpless." In the sick room, as Woolf scholar Jane Marcus has pointed out, the Victorian woman could exert a power denied her in the world outside the home, a world where even a healthy woman might often feel "help-less."[20] Literary critic Kimberly Coates has sug-gested that Woolf's *On Being Ill* may repudiate her mother's "art of nursing" in favor of the imaginative possibilities of the "art of being ill."[21] Although Woolf probably did not specifically recall *Notes from Sick Rooms* when she was writing *On Being Ill*, we do know that her mother was very much on her mind as she began to write *To the Lighthouse*. We know, for example, that she was carrying her 1905 Cornwall diary with her as she began to work on the novel because she wrote to Vita Sackville-West that she may have left it at her house, or perhaps at her sister Vanessa's. Because it lets us hear the voice of the mother who Woolf tells us "obsessed" her until she wrote *To the Lighthouse*, *Notes from Sick Rooms* is therefore an enlightening text to read with *On Being Ill*, an important piece of nursing history, a guide for care givers today, and also a fascinating docu-ment in the biography of one of the twentieth cen-tury's greatest novelists.

MARK HUSSEY
JULY 28, 2012

NOTES

Notes from Sick Rooms by Mrs. Leslie Stephen was published by Smith, Elder & Co., London, 1883. (George Smith, the publisher of Charlotte Brontë, was a close friend of Leslie Stephen.) An edition introduced by Constance Hunting was published by Puckerbrush Press, Orono, Maine, in 1980. *Notes* is also included in *Julia Duckworth Stephen, Stories for Children, Essays for Adults*, edited by Diane F. Gillespie and Elizabeth Steele, published by Syracuse University Press in 1987.

1. Virginia Woolf, "A Sketch of the Past," *Moments of Being*, ed. Jeanne Schulkind, San Diego: Harcourt, 1985 ["Sketch"], 81.
2. Examples can be found in Julia Margaret Cameron, *Victorian Photographs of Famous Men & Fair Women* (1926), London: Hogarth Press, 1973.
3. *Sir Leslie Stephen's Mausoleum Book*, with an introduction by Alan Bell, Oxford: Clarendon, 1977 [*Mausoleum*], 40. Within two weeks of his wife's death, Leslie Stephen began a long account of their marriage addressed to her children. It became known within the family as "The Mausoleum Book."
4. Letter to Charles Eliot Norton, 4 March 1878, *Selected Letters of Leslie Stephen*, Vol. I: 1864-1882, ed. John W. Bicknell, Columbus: Ohio State University Press, 1996 [Bicknell], 230.
5. *Mausoleum*, 27.
6. "Sketch," 83.
7. Vanessa Bell, *Notes on Virginia's Childhood*, New York: Frank Hallman, 1974 [Bell], unpaginated.
8. Julia Stephen's published and unpublished writings are found in *Julia Duckworth Stephen, Stories for Children, Essays for Adults*, ed. Diane F. Gillespie and Elizabeth Steele, Syracuse: Syracuse University

Press, 1987 [Gillespie and Steele]. Anyone writing on Julia Stephen must, as I am, be indebted to this volume.

9. Virginia Woolf, *A Passionate Apprentice: The Early Journals, 1897-1909*, ed. Mitchell A. Leaska, San Diego: Harcourt, 1990, 285.

10. "Sketch," 131.

11. See Panthea Reid, "Appendix A: Virginia's Childhood and Her Grandmother's Letters," *Art and Affection: A Life of Virginia Woolf*, New York: Oxford University Press, 1996, 458.

12. *Mausoleum*, 40.

13. *The Nursing Record & Hospital World* (1 May 1897), http://tiny.cc/5pu8iw, 18 August 2012.

14. *Mausoleum*, 40.

15. Florence Nightingale, *Notes on Nursing: What it is and what it is not* (1859), New York: Dover, 1969, 3.

16. "Agnostic Women," in Gillespie and Steele, 243.

17. *The Flight of the Mind: The Letters of Virginia Woolf*, Vol. I: 1888-1912, ed. Nigel Nicolson and Joanne Trautmann, London: Hogarth Press, 1975, 247-266.

18. Winifred Holtby, *Virginia Woolf*, London: Wishart, 1932, 12-13.

19. *The Diary of Virginia Woolf*, Vol. III, ed. Anne Olivier Bell, Hogarth Press, 1980, 21 December 1925, 58.

20. Jane Marcus, "Virginia Woolf and Her Violin: Mothering, Madness and Music," *Virginia Woolf and the Languages of Patriarchy*, Bloomington: Indiana University Press, 1987, 97.

21. Kimberly Engdahl Coates, "Phantoms, Fancy (And) Symptoms: Virginia Woolf and the Art of Being Ill," *Woolf Studies Annual*, 18 (2011), 1-28.

NOTES FROM SICK ROOMS

PREFACE

My experience both as nurse and as patient has been too limited to justify me in adding to the existing stock of notes upon nursing, were it not that I have taken pains to note down things which have come under my actual observation, either as giving relief, or causing discomfort to the sufferer. I must leave much that is obvious unsaid, and I am aware that I say much which seems too obvious to require saying.

My excuse must be that I have wished to keep strictly to what I have learnt, or unlearnt, in sick rooms. I do not pretend to lay down any large rules as to nursing, but I wish to point out how some of the many disagreeable circumstances attendant upon illness may be diminished or removed. I have been able to watch the nursing of experienced hospital nurses, and I have been with those who had the highest characters for efficiency, and with those who were neither trained nor efficient, but who yet had something to teach.

I have also had the actual nursing of some cases, and have suffered too much from my own shortcomings not to wish to turn them to account for others.

I have often wondered why it is considered a proof of virtue in anyone to become a nurse. The ordinary relations between the sick and the well are far easier and pleasanter than between the well and the well.

There are no doubt people to whom the sight of physical suffering is so distasteful as to turn a sick room into a real Chamber of Horrors for them. That such unlucky persons should ever have authority in a sick room ought to be an impossibility; but if by some unlucky chance they ever have, we should surely reserve our pity for the unfortunate invalids in their charge.

Illness has, or ought to have, much of the levelling power of death. We forget, or at all events cease to dwell on, the unfavourable sides to a character when death has claimed its owner, and in illness we can afford to ignore the details which in health make familiar intercourse difficult.

The ways in which our friends dress, bring up their children, or spend their money, are apt to cause disagreement more or less marked between us when there is no thought of suffering or loss; but the moment we are threatened by either, how slight such matters seem! We can contemplate without irritation the vivid fringe of hair when the head which it disfigures is aching and fevered; and we feel equal to allowing the spoilt children to put their feet in the 'crystal butter-boat,' like the never-to-be-forgotten little boy of our childhood, if it will give any pleasure to the over indulgent mother who is racked with pain.

NURSING INSTINCT

A NURSE'S LIFE is certainly not a dull one, and the more skilful the nurse the less dull she will be. The more she cultivates the *art* of nursing, the more enjoyment she will get, and the same may be said of the patient. The art of being ill is no easy one to learn, but it is practised to perfection by many of the greatest sufferers.

The greatest sufferer is by no means the worst patient, and to give relief, even if it be only temporary, to such patients is perhaps a greater pleasure than can be found in the performance of any other duty.

It ought to be quite immaterial to a nurse whom she is nursing. I have often heard it urged against trained nurses that they look upon their patients as *cases*. If to look on patients as a case is to feel indifference towards them, then the charge is indeed a reproof; but assuming that the nurse is not indifferent, how should she look on her patient but as a case; and further, why should she?

The genuine love of her 'case' and not of the individual patient seems to me the sign of the true nursing instinct.

It would be hard if those who were specially charming, or whose antecedents interested, were alone to be tenderly nursed. Every nurse, whether trained or amateur, should look on her patient as a 'case,' nursing with the same undeviating tenderness and watchful care the entire stranger, the unsympathetic friend, or the one who is nearest and dearest.

In most cases of illness nursed at home, even if there be a trained nurse, there is generally some member of the family watching and helping—more often hindering the work of the sick room.

Much may be done by such helpers to make the lives of both patient and nurse easier and brighter; but unless such outsiders help with skill and tact, as well as with zeal, their presence in the sick room is dreaded instead of desired.

To avoid confusion I have used the word 'nurse,' but many of the little hints which I have noted down are for such watchers. One imperative duty of all those in attendance on the sick is that they should be cheerful; not an elaborate, forced cheerfulness, but a quiet brightness which makes their presence a cheer and not an oppression. It may seem difficult to follow this advice, but it is not. Cheerfulness is a habit, and no one should venture to attend the sick who wears a gloomy face. The atmosphere of the sick room should be cheerful and peaceful. Domestic disturbances, money matters, worries, and discussions of all kinds should be kept away.

LYING

THERE CAN BE no half dealing in such matters; hints and whispers are worse than the whole truth. There is no limit to a sick person's imagination, and this is a fact which is too often ignored, even by the tenderest friends. The answers, 'Oh, it is nothing,' 'Don't worry yourself,' when suspicion is once aroused, are enough to fret the unfortunate patient into a fever. She will torture herself with suspicion of every possible calamity, and at last, when she has nerved herself to insist on being told, her unconscious tormentor discloses the fact that one of the pipes has burst!

If trouble should come, and it is important that the invalid should be kept in ignorance, her watchers must make peace with their consciences as best they can; and if questions are asked, they must 'lie freely.'

CRUMBS

AMONG THE NUMBER of small evils which haunt illness, the greatest, in the misery which it can cause, though the smallest in size, is crumbs. The origin of most things has been decided on, but the origin of crumbs in bed has never excited sufficient attention among the scientific world, though it is a problem which has tormented many a weary sufferer. I will forbear to give my own explanation, which would be neither scientific nor orthodox, and will merely beg that their evil existence may be recognised and, as far as human nature allows, guarded against. The torment of crumbs should be stamped out of the sick bed as if it were the Colorado beetle in a potato field. Anyone who has been ill will at once take her precautions, feeble though they will prove. She will have a napkin under her chin, stretch her neck out of bed, eat in the most uncomfortable way, and watch that no crumbs get into the folds of her night-dress or jacket. When she lies back in bed, in the vain hope that she may have baffled the enemy, he is before her: a sharp crumb is buried in her back, and grains of sand seem sticking to her toes. If the patient is able to get up and have her bed made, when she returns to it she will find the crumbs are waiting for her. The housemaid will protest that the sheets were shaken, and the nurse that she swept out the crumbs, but there they are, and there they will remain unless the nurse determines to conquer them. To do this she must first believe in them, and there are few assertions that are met with such incredulity as the one—I have crumbs in my bed. After every meal the nurse should put her hand into the bed and feel for the crumbs. When the bed is made, the nurse and housemaid must not content themselves with shaking or sweeping. The tiny crumbs stick in the sheets, and the nurse must patiently take each crumb out; if there are many very small ones, she must even wet her fingers, and get the crumbs to stick to them. The patient's night-clothes must be searched; crumbs lurk in each tiny fold or frill. They go up the sleeve of the night-gown, and if the patient is in bed when the search is going on, her arms should hang out of bed, so that the crumbs which are certain to be there may be induced to fall down. When crumbs are banished—that is to say, temporarily, for with each meal they return, and for this the nurse must make up her mind—she must see that there are no rucks in the bed-sheets. A very good way of avoiding these is to pin the lower sheet firmly down on the mattress with nursery pins, first stretching the sheet smoothly and straightly over the mattress.

BED

MANY PEOPLE ARE not aware of the importance of putting on a sheet *straight*, but if it is not, it will certainly drag, and if pinned it will probably tear. The blankets should be put on lightly, one by one, not two or three at a time. There is an appreciable difference in the way in which coverings are laid upon people. Each covering should be laid on straight and smooth; no pulling straight should be done afterwards. If the patient is in bed when her

bed is made, the lower sheet should be half rolled
up and laid on the edge; the patient should then be
lifted over the roll on to the fresh sheet, half of
which has been spread over half of the bed. The old
sheet can easily be pulled away, and when the new
one is unrolled it can at once be tucked in and
pinned if required. The upper sheet is rolled or
folded breadth-ways and laid under the blankets,
beginning at the feet; it is then quickly drawn up
and the old one removed, the blankets not being dis-
turbed. All blankets and quilts should be so
arranged as not to drag and not to slip; any extra
covering which is required only over the feet should
not drag down to be pulled off by each movement of
the patient, or by a careless passer by; it should be
supported on a towel-horse unless there is a good
footboard to the bed. If there is not a good footboard, it is well to improvise one by putting a plain
deal board at the end of the bed between the mattress and the bars, as the legs of a towel-horse or a
chair are very liable to be kicked by passers by, and
the bed gets shaken, a thing much to be avoided.

If an eider-down quilt is wanted, it should be
pinned with American safety pins on to the top
covering.

A sick bed is apt to become close and unpleasant, but the nurse may refresh it without chilling the
patient if she raises the top sheet, with the coverings
resting on it, three or four times, thus fanning the
bed and causing the patient no fatigue or chill. An
invalid can air her own bed in this way if she can
raise her knees; she need then only lift the outer
edge of the sheet up with her hand and raise one
knee up and down; but this of course requires some
strength, and the bed will be more effectually aired
by some one standing by the side of it.

Some people think that the whole comfort of a
bed depends on its pillows, and I am not sure that
they are not right. Certainly a hard or a pappy pillow will make an otherwise comfortable bed a most
unresting one. Everyone has their own way of
arranging their pillows: some like them smooth and
straight, while others twist and turn them till it
seems as if no head could find rest. The nurse must
find out which way her patient prefers before
attempting to arrange the pillows. I have often seen
a sick person tormented by the over zealous nurse
seizing the pillow and altering what certainly
seemed a most uncomfortable arrangement, but one
which was in fact exactly suited to the patient's

needs, and only attained after many struggles. The
nurse must be always ready to turn the pillow when
wanted; she can do this without fatiguing the
patient by placing one hand at the back of the sick
person's head, while with the other she quickly
turns the pillow and slips it back into its place. I say
hand advisedly. The palm hollowed inwards a little
should be used. Nurses very often make use of two
fingers, which, when well pressed in at the back of
the head, make the turning of pillows a very tortur-
ing process. Where no second pillow is at hand, and
the patient wishes to have her head higher, she can
make a comfortable change for herself by doubling
the corner of the pillow back or under her cheek;
but no nurse can attempt such an arrangement, as it
may be such an uncomfortable one, that it is only by
the patient's own hand and cheek that the proper
curve can be made.

WATERPROOF

IF A WATERPROOF sheet is necessary, the best way
to make the bed is as follows: the bed having been
made as usual, with a good blanket under the lower
sheet, the waterproof should be laid on it, over the
waterproof a blanket, and again over the blanket a

sheet; these should not be tucked in. When the waterproof is no longer wanted, the top sheet, blanket, and waterproof can all be drawn away from under the patient, who will find herself on a clean, freshly-made bed.

The shorter time that a waterproof can be kept under a patient the better; the smell and heat cause much discomfort, and with a good under-blanket the mattress will seldom come to grief. Nurses are very apt to exaggerate the necessity for a waterproof, and are unwilling to believe in the restlessness and discomfort created by one. Economy is a great virtue in a nurse, for all illness, however slight, involves expense; but the virtue may be carried to excess.

There are, I believe, many people who would rather suffer a great deal of discomfort than swell their washing bill; and if the nurse should find this to be the case, she must do all she can, while keeping the patient sweet and fresh, to save expense. Nothing can do a sick person more harm than to worry over accounts and expenses, and if the patient should be one of those notable house-wives to whom any exceeding of a certain sum is absolute misery, her peculiarity in this as in all other respects during illness should be respected. If, however, the nurse has not got to deal with such a patient, but may secure the *luxuries* of cleanliness, I would counsel her to have as much clean linen and as many clean clothes as she can lay hands on.

It is, as far as I have been able to judge, an invariable rule among nurses that when only one clean sheet is used, the clean one should be placed on the top, and the one that was on the top should be placed below.

The obvious reason for doing this is, that the top sheet is the one that is seen, and therefore should have a glossy freshness. The obvious reason against it is that the bottom sheet is the most felt, and therefore, in the interest of the patient's comfort, I would beg that whenever one clean sheet only is put on, it may be the one on which the patient has to lie. I am quite aware that the top sheet is only *tumbled*, not soiled; but it is that very tumbling, that want of smoothness and freshness, that makes a long stay in bed so trying. And if, as we take for granted, the top sheet *is* only tumbled, the doctor can surely be allowed the sight of it. Unless the patient be a Mrs. Skelton, she will prefer to have her comfort consulted rather than her appearance.

HANDKERCHIEFS

IF CRUMBS ARE the most tenacious inhabitants of a bed, handkerchiefs may be considered as the most transitory; they disappear mysteriously, although they have been invariably placed under the pillow. To obviate a little the perpetual game of hunt the handkerchief, it is well that the patient should be provided with two handkerchiefs—one placed under each end of the pillow. If the invalid should wear a bed jacket, it should be furnished with pockets. With regard to jackets, I would advise that they should be made with large armholes and sleeves, sufficiently large to allow of the night-gown sleeve passing under with ease. There should be no thick frilling or trimming at the throat; although in the hand such jackets look pretty and becoming, they are hot and uncomfortable to wear, and as the frills soon turn in and get untidy, in a short time they do not even look well.

WASHING

THERE IS NO part of nursing more troublesome, more necessary, or more to be deplored, than washing. We know that there are many people who have

a perfect mania for washing. Speaking to such
invalids, I would entreat them to repress their desire
for soap and water as if it were for gin; to be content
with a small wash every day, and not to torment
themselves with the idea that, unless they are
washed all over every day in the most scrupulous
manner, they must be dirty. The nurse, however,
has not come to root up her patient's theories, but to
carry them out as far as may be in accordance with
the patient's well-doing. This is often not very easy;
but a very thorough washing may be done without
risk of chill, and with comparatively little fatigue, if
the nurse manages well.

All that is required for washing should be ready
at hand—hot and cold water, a bath-thermometer,
and plenty of warm towels; an old flannel dressing-
gown; a spare blanket should also be at hand. Before
attempting to uncover her patient, the nurse must be
certain that she has all she can possibly want; there
should be no moving to and fro, no coming into the
room, and no delays when the work of washing has
once begun.

The patient must of course be washed piecemeal;
the uncovered part must be covered with a loose
flannel which has been warmed, and the washing and

drying must be done under this flannel whenever it is practicable.

Each part should be well dried, and covered with something that will not slip off—if the clothes cannot at once be put on—before the rest of the washing is begun. A little vinegar, eau de Cologne, or rose water, makes washing more refreshing, and eau de Cologne prevents a chill. The towels, which should all be well warmed, should not be scorching. The skin is very sensitive after washing, and the towel should be of an equable warmth, with no very hot bits, and should be given gently; the sudden giving of a towel and flapping the air against the patient's wet skin produces an icy chill, a fact of which nurses are too often unconscious. If there are two attendants while washing is going on, one should busy herself with the towels, moving them in front of the fire, so that every part is well warmed while none is scorching. If the nurse is single-handed, she should have her towels warming at a little distance from the fire some time before wash-ing begins, and should turn them when she begins. If, by a chance, she finds any part of a towel has become too hot—and she should always pass her hand rapidly over the towels before using them—a quick shake out while the patient remains covered would make the towel of a comfortable temperature.

When there is no fire a hot foot-warmer, round which the towels can be wrapped, does almost as well.

BATH

IN GIVING A bath the same course must be pursued in a great measure; but if the patient has to be carried into the bath, the nurse must be very careful to lower her gently into the bath. In bathing a helpless patient it will be found almost imperative to have two attendants. The patient's feet should be allowed to feel the water first, and the water should be moved by the hand of the nurse, while the patient is being placed in the bath, so that it laps up to the patient's body, and that she avoids all shock. Being lifted into a bath causes great nervousness, far greater than the bystanders can credit; and the nurse should make her patient's mind as much at rest as she can, not only by telling her the exact temperature of the water, but by letting her feel it with her fingers before she is put in. When lifted out, a large warm sheet should be ready with which at once the patient is covered; she must then be carried to a sofa, on which must be spread a warm blanket; on this the patient lies, and in it she is wrapped; the sheet which has taken off the first wet is removed from under the blanket, and the patient is dried thoroughly with warm towels. A patient bathed in this way should feel little fatigue; but the bathing and drying must be done in silence. The useless remarks in which attendants indulge are absolutely injurious to sick people. The 'All right,' 'Oh, here it is,' 'Wait a moment,' irritate and take away all the refreshment which the bath would have given.

The nurse must be very careful not to hurt by rubbing or by soaping any scratch or sore place that a patient may have. The hurt may seem insignificant, but nothing is small in illness, and a little scratch well soaped will set up a very considerable 'raw,' and effectually prevent a nervous patient from sleeping. The nurse should be careful to keep her hands smooth and her nails short; the lovely filbert nails which are the pride of many are very literal 'thorns in the flesh' of the unlucky patient, who derives no consolation from the assurance given by the nurse, 'You can't feel a pin, ma'am, for my fingers are there.'

When the hands are washed, the basin should be held below the hand, so that the water may drip down, not run up the sleeve, as is often the case. If by chance the sleeve should get wet, a piece of cotton wool should be placed between the wetted part and the arm, and the wet spot should be well sprinkled with eau de Cologne. If the bed should be slightly wetted, eau de Cologne sprinkled on it will prevent a chill; but if there is much wet, and it is impossible to change the sheet, a hot iron should be passed up and down the wet part, which will soon dry. In doing this extreme care must be taken not only that the patient should not be burnt, but that she should herself feel assured that such precautions have been taken that she cannot be burnt.

It is a great refreshment to sick people to have their feet washed, and no part of the body can be washed more safely and with less fatigue to the patient. A warm flannel must be put under the foot, which should hang a little over the side of the bed, the foot-tub or basin must be just below, and the foot can thus be soaped and sponged easily and effectually.

Each foot must be washed separately, and, as the sponge is removed, must be wrapped in a warm flannel and dried with warm towels. In cases of advanced chest disease, the patient will probably be very much afraid of having her feet washed; but if the nurse can persuade her to have them done, she will reap even greater advantage than other patients, for in such diseases a thick dry skin forms over the foot, causing intolerable heat and irritation. When actual washing is not required, refreshment will be found in rubbing eau de Cologne over the feet and between the toes.

HAIR

IN DOING THE invalid's hair, the nurse would do well to use at first only a comb with large teeth, or, if she has not got one, only to use the large teeth of an ordinary comb. She should hold the hair near the roots with one hand, so that the patient should not suffer if a tangled part has to be combed out. The hair should be lightly touched, the head being kept steady, not pulled from one side to the other, as is often done.

The nurse should be careful to see *where* her brush goes. It is an absurd but unpleasant fact, that an invalid's eyebrows often get quite as much of the brush as her hair. The nurse should always clear the brush of loose hairs before using it. Few things are more aggravating than to have a long hair brought slowly over the face each time the brush comes round.

Hairs are not so bad as crumbs, but they are very tormenting bed-fellows, and there is little excuse for any nurse who, after brushing the patient's hair, allows any stray hairs to remain on the night-dress or bed-clothes.

When the bed-pan is required the nurse should not oblige the patient to raise herself twice; she should slip the pan at once into the proper position, and when she removes it she can at the same time straighten down the patient's clothes.

If the invalid should be very weak and nervous, a small waterproof and towel can be kept under the bed-pan; these can be placed at the same time as the pan itself. Burnt vinegar is the most pleasant of scented disinfectants. An old jam-pot with vinegar in it, into which one or two live coals are dropped, is the safest way of using it. The scent of the vinegar, unless the patient objects to it, is far more healthy then ruban de Bruges, or pastilles. Sanitas is an admirable purifier. When used in a little squirt, it will soon remove all unpleasantness; it is most refreshing on the clothes and inside the bed. Boracic acid is an admirable deodoriser; if some of the crystals dissolved in water are placed in the utensil before it is used, no unpleasantness will be perceived, and, as it is colourless and without smell, it is preferable to either Condy or carbolic acid.

AIR

SUCH GREAT AUTHORITIES have written on ventilation, that I need only say that there is no danger in having a thorough draught through a sick room each day, provided that the patient is not only thoroughly well wrapped up while the windows are open, but for some time after they are shut, and that the coverings are only removed by degrees.

Candle smoke is one of the most unpleasant smells in a sick room, and it is so constantly breathed by invalids, even when they have careful and considerate nurses, that I will venture to assert emphatically that there is only one way in which the smoke can be destroyed with absolute certainty— that is, by dabbing the wick with a spill, paper cutter, or any flat light thing that may be at hand.[1] The

1 Since writing the above, a friend has sent me a delightful pair of snuffers, the only ones I have ever seen that quench the flame without producing smoke: they are flat instead of box-shaped, and neither cut nor crush the wick, while they effectually prevent any smell.

wick can be raised the moment the flame is out, and the candle will not be spoiled. Blowing a candle out upwards, or blowing it out while it is held up the chimney, are good ways, but not infallible. An extinguisher is the worst of all, as it imprisons the smoke, which either discharges itself by degrees, thus lengthening out the torment, or remains in the extinguisher till the candle is again wanted, and then escapes, and the last state is without doubt worse than the first. Night-lights should be dabbed out too, for they have a most unpleasant smell; they should never be put in the fire; there is no smell more offensive than that of grease burning.

LIGHT

MANY INVALIDS OBJECT to a light in the room at night. When this is the case, the nurse should dispense, if possible, with one. It is more often possible than nurses are willing to think. Candles and matches must, of course, be at hand, and it is well to have a light in the next room or passage; but if a patient wishes her room to be dark, the nurse should endeavour to make it so.

When a light is required, it should be skilfully shaded. By skilful shading I mean not only that the light itself should be shaded, but that its reflection must be hidden as much as possible from the eyes of the sick person.

I have seen a candle shade carefully arranged by a kind and skilful nurse so as completely to hide the actual candle, but she ignored the fact that the light was reflected by a mirror just behind it. A night-light is often put in a basin for safety and shade, but a beautiful globe of light will be reflected on the ceiling, the light of the little lamp being increased tenfold by the glazed china. Daylight has to be shaded with equal care. If the blinds and curtains are drawn, the nurse must see that there is no crack left open. A slant gleam of light is more trying than the broad shaft which would come if the curtains were not closed.

Wherever lights are placed the nurse must be careful that they are not near anything which can suggest the idea of danger to the patient's mind. One of the many terrors which haunt the helpless is that of being burnt in their beds. Distances do not appear the same to those up and those in bed. What may be obviously safe to a person standing up, looks perilously close to one in bed; and the nurse must not argue the point, but must either move the light, or, if that cannot be, she must *prove* to the patient's own satisfaction that there is no danger.

One of the many mistakes into which nurses fall is that of persuading patients, or at least trying to persuade them (for we know how seldom people well or ill *are* persuaded). A sick person will often give in from sheer fatigue; but she remains unconvinced, and her mind is not at rest; she goes over and over her reasons and the nurse's, and worries herself over a thing of small importance, because she does not like to reopen the discussion. I would impress on all nurses strongly that, as far as lies in their power, they should keep their patient's mind at rest. They cannot control the disturbing influences which find their way into the sick room, nor can they overcome all the varied miseries which beset the sick brain; but some of these miseries they can soothe, and they can and should always be careful not to cause any themselves.

FANCIES

INVALIDS' FANCIES SEEM, and often are, absurd; but arguing will not dissipate them; it will only increase them, as the patient will hide what she feels, and so increase her mental discomfort—a sure way of augmenting her physical suffering. One of the many rewards that come to a careful and considerate nurse is that the patient's fancies are not absurd. If the invalid knows that her nurse has undertaken to see that a thing is right, she will have an easy mind about it, and will not worry the nurse with useless questions and suggestions.

There are, of course, patients who, without meaning to be exacting, are so delicately organised, or whose senses have become so acute through suffering, that they can detect a draught or a smell where even careful and discerning nurses can find neither. The nurse must, therefore, not deny that the evil exists; a door or a window may have been opened without her knowledge, and the current of air may be felt by the sick though not by the well. Something may have been dropped on the kitchen fire, or there may be some minute escape of gas which is imperceptible to all but the invalid. The nurse must remove these evils should they exist, and thoroughly investigate the evil real or fancied. Cold cannot be taken through the imagination; but a nervous dread of chill can make a sick person thoroughly wretched, and one of the chief duties of a nurse is to make her patient thoroughly comfortable in mind and body.

If the patient be well enough to be left for any time she should always have a bell, and any small thing that she is likely to want in a hurry, close by her. The nurse should never leave her patient hastily, but wait to be certain that all the things are there, and that the invalid has said all she wants. The mind moves slowly to expression in illness, and the feeling that the words are impatiently waited for takes away the power to utter them.

A nurse, especially if she be an amateur, will find it useful to keep a written record of the events of the sick room—the hours at which food and medicine are taken, any variation of temperature or symptoms, the amount of sleep that the patient has had, &c. The monotony of a sick room is very great. Anyone who tries to remember in their order the small events which make up the invalid's day will be astonished to find how perplexed she is when any doubt is thrown on her statement. The doctor is very glad to have the diary of a careful watcher. Such symptoms as flushings, restlessness, excitement, and the hours

at which they occur, are important features in illness, but at the time of the doctor's visit the nurse
is nevertheless very apt to forget them, unless they
have been noted down.

VISITS

IT IS A truism that one's friends are one's greatest
enemies, but in illness it is a very painful fact; and
the number of ways which kind people find of tormenting each other would be amusing were it not
so painful. Most invalids have some hour when
they may be visited, but it is in vain that they
impress this fact on their friends. Day after day the
unwelcome announcement is made that so and so
knows she is too early but she will wait. The
invalid hurries through her meal or her dressing,
or whatever she may be about, and so is quite unfit
to enjoy her friend's visit when it is paid.

Visitors have an uncomfortable habit of apolo-
gising for their visits. The invalid has, no doubt,
much she wishes to say and to hear, and the time for
the visit is short; it is therefore extremely irritating
to have it made shorter by visitors who keep on
assuring her that they won't stay a minute, and they
don't mean to talk, &c. There is a delusion under

which most visitors to an invalid labour—that all illness affects either the brain or the hearing. It is impossible otherwise to account for the patronising cheerfulness and the peculiar distinctness of utterance which such visitors affect. We are reminded irresistibly of the excellent Mrs. Peckaby, who spoke broken English in order to make herself understood by M. Baptiste.

Visitors should come straight into the sick room; there should be no delay and whispering outside after they have been announced; they should not begin to talk till they are well within eye and ear range of the sick person. The habit of coming half in, of beginning to speak while still at the door, and still worse speaking while holding the door open (this practice is the almost invariable one of servants bringing a message, and should be checked by the nurse), all show that the visitors had far better keep away till their friends are well. If the patient is asleep and a visitor comes in, she should go away instantly, not stand and gaze till the invalid wakes, as she invariably does, with a start.

The patient's bed should never be sat upon nor held. Such remarks may seem uncalled for but very little experience in a sick room will convince anyone that they are not. Hurried visits are much to be discouraged. An invalid would often prefer not to see her greatest friend than to feel that the visit is such a gasp; no pleasant talk can be heard, no refreshing sight of each other enjoyed.

The nurse must take it upon herself to turn away visitors. If it is difficult and disagreeable to her to do it, she must remember that it is far more difficult and unpleasant for the patient herself, who probably would not have the courage to tell her friends to go, though she will be very thankful if her nurse does.

NOISES

ALL MOVEMENTS IN the sick room should be quiet. I do not mean in the matter of banging doors and creaking footsteps, for people who are so noisy have no business in a sick room.

Nurses or visitors to a sick room should be quiet and steady in all their movements; they should not start up from their seat, however hurriedly they may be required; the rustle of clothes, the dropping of things off a lap, and the search for them afterwards, make the invalid regret that she caused such disturbance.

When evening draws on, the nurse should see that she has all the things in readiness that her patient can possibly require. She should not only have the food and medicines which are to be taken during the night, but she should see that the kettle is full, that she has matches, wood, and coal, a spare candle or two, plenty of water, and that materials for making poultices are at hand. It is a common experience how often illness takes a turn or a new form in the night; and the nurse should be provided with all ordinary remedies so as to be able to lose no time in applying them. Nothing should have to be sent for late. There should be no bustle or noise in the sick room. As night approaches the room should become gradually still. The fire must be arranged early, for no noise is more exasperating than the scraping up of cinders, or the raking out of coals. In short, the room should be so gently hushed that the patient should feel able to drop off to sleep at any moment, and not lose her one chance of rest, perhaps, from the sense that there is something disturbing still to be done. A night nurse should sit near the fire so as to keep her hands warm, as much for her patient's sake as her own. The touch of a cold hand will rouse a person thoroughly; and though the patient may be awake, the nurse's object is to soothe her off to sleep as soon as may be. A pair of housemaid's gloves ought to lie by the coals, which can then be put on the fire without risk of disturbing the patient or of soiling the nurse's hands.

FEEDING

IF FOOD HAS to be given at night, the heating of it or other preparation should, if possible, take place in the next room to the patient's. If this cannot be, the nurse should be very quiet about it, and, when prepared, she should not offer it to her patient, except in cases of excessive weakness, unless she is quite sure that her patient is really awake.

It is one of the vagaries of illness that a sick person, who has been unable to sleep all night, will drop off the moment after she has asked for her meal. There would seem to be something in the knowledge that something is being actually prepared for their relief, which rests the mind and makes the sufferer go to sleep. When this is the case, however troublesome it may be, the nurse must make up her mind to let the food remain untouched, and to prepare fresh the next time it is asked for. The food should be given in a regular, monotonous way, so that the patient is as little roused as possible.

A spirit lamp is invaluable for heating food or boiling water; it should be placed on a marble stand or table, if possible, as the spirit is constantly upset, and though the flame is soon extinguished and not very harmful, the flame rouses and alarms the invalid.

If the patient likes being read to at night, the reader's voice must be clear and loud enough for each word to be heard without effort. If the patient should fall asleep while the reading is going on, the reader must on no account stop, but must go on reading for some time in the same tone, and then gradually allow her voice to die away.

When an illness has gone on for some time the sick person becomes very weary of the things which surround her. She has looked at all the pictures which hang on the walls, and at the patterns which ornament or disfigure the paper, till she can bear them no longer. The nurse cannot, of course, alter all these things, but she can give a certain change to the aspect of the room. A looking-glass so placed that it can reflect the sky and trees, or, if the sufferer is in London, some portion of the street, will be a refreshment to the eyes which have for long not pierced beyond the narrow boundary of the sick room.

Plants and flowers should be placed so as to show their best shape and colour to the invalid's eye, and in such a position as to be seen by her easily without any exertion. Many people are worried by the sight of a thing placed crookedly, and a nervous patient will dread the appearance of anything placed near the edge of the table. She will go through in imagination the crash which will follow if the book or vase is swept down by a passer by.

When a message has to be given or a note written, the nurse or friend should endeavour to carry out the sick person's wishes as quickly as possible. The most patient of invalids cannot overcome a feeling of disappointment if told that what they have begged may be done at once, has been put off, or will be done in good time. In the dulness of an invalid's life small trifles become important; and although the note which had to be sent may have been of no great moment, the invalid has probably been counting on the answer, and may very likely another time make an effort to write herself rather than be kept in suspense.

DRESSING

WHEN THE PATIENT can be dressed and put on a sofa, the nurse must gather the patient's sleeves up in her hand, so that the arm may pass in without difficulty.

All clothes should be warmed before being put on, and all should be put on straight, not dragged straight afterwards. The first getting up is made miserable to the convalescent by her clothes; every movement rucks them up, and she is not yet strong enough to stand up and give them a shake down.

The nurse must always be ready to pull down the patient's clothes, and she must begin with the flannel, or whatever garment the patient wears next her skin, and work outwards, not, as is almost invariably done, begin by the petticoat, and so leave off where she should have begun. Care must be taken not to pull the clothes down too tight, or they will drag at the throat, which is most uncomfortable.

I have tried in the foregoing pages to note down some of the ordinary duties of a nurse; I have tried to point out how many little details there are in the every day-work of the sick room which can hardly be called nursing, and yet which, if badly performed or neglected, materially affect the patient's comfort, perhaps even retard her recovery.

COOKING

I NOW WISH to add a few words about various remedies and the ways of making use of them in various forms of illness. I am quite aware that I must leave much unsaid that ought to be said, but I wish only to give my own experience, and to tell of remedies that I have found useful, or useless, in such cases of illness as I have had the opportunity of watching. As all nurses should know something of cooking, and be ready to prepare food for their patient, I will begin with the invalid's food. The nurse must of course see all the food before it is given to her patient, even when she does not give it herself. Beef-tea often comes from the kitchen with a fair coating of grease. The nurse can remove this by floating little bits of whitey-brown paper on the surface, which will blot up the grease in a very few seconds. As the cup will probably smell greasy and look messy, the nurse should pour the hot beef-tea into a clean hot cup which she should have ready. If the beef-tea should be thick, the nurse should strain it through a piece of muslin which she has wetted in cold water. After doing this, she will have to warm up the beef-tea on her spirit lamp.

One or two extra cups, glasses, and spoons, a bowl, and clean cloth should always be at hand. The best feeding cups are of glass, which are easily cleaned with a baby's bottle brush. A certain variety may be made in beef-tea, of which patients are certain to weary, by mixing veal with the beef.

The best beef-tea is made of two or three pounds of freshly killed beefsteak, with an equal quantity of veal. The meat must be cut up into dice, all fat and skin being removed, and placed in a jar with a little salt, and enough water to cover the meat. This jar, which must have either a lid or a thick cloth tied over the top, is then placed in a saucepan of water on the fire and left to stew. In three hours a cup of strong beef-tea is procured; but it is better to let the whole quantity be made and allowed to get cold; the fat can then be cleared off, and the beef-tea, which is then jelly, can be warmed as it is required. If a large quantity is made at once, it must be well boiled up every day or it will turn sour. The nurse and patient must remember that the strongest beef-tea does not produce a stiff jelly. Unless a little of the shin of beef or knuckle of veal is put in, a jelly of any consistency cannot be got. This must be done if the invalid likes sometimes to have jelly instead of soup, and the beef-tea must be well reduced or the jelly will be insipid.

Reducing simply means letting the beef-tea boil away; you reduce the quantity but not the quality. This explanation seems superfluous, but I have known a good nurse 'reduce' beef-tea by adding water to it. The nurse must remember that when gravy or broth is much reduced it does not require salt. A patient suffering from soreness of the mouth will often complain that too much salt has been put in the beef-tea, and will be silenced by the answer that there is none. If the patient is suffering in this way, her food must not be much reduced, for the increased strength produces increased saltness. If the invalid has to be fed, the meat must be cut up most carefully, the patient's tastes being scrupulously observed. The mouthfuls given must be of medium size; people often imagine that little scraps will tempt a patient, but the fact is that very tiny mouthfuls weary the patient of her food long before she has eaten all she should. The nurse must never touch the patient's food with her hands, and must have perfectly clean hands before she begins to feed the invalid; she should never blow anything that is hot.

FOOD

WHEN HELPING THE patient to eat or drink, the nurse should support the head with her hand and tilt the cup or glass gently, but sufficiently. It is most aggravating to be able only to sip when you want a refreshing draught.

Beef-tea may be thickened with Groult's tapioca, sufficient being put in to make the soup of a pleasant consistency; the tapioca must be stirred in while the soup is boiling. Arrowroot can be put in soup in the same way, and is useful when the bowels are relaxed. Macaroni boiled in gravy is nourishing, and can be taken with meat when vegetables are either not allowed or not liked. The macaroni must be well stirred while cooking in the gravy, or it will not be soft, although it may have been cooking a long time.

If vegetables are taken, they should be removed from the room at once, as any green vegetables have an unpleasant smell.

In cases of nausea, cold food will be found far more palatable than hot; cold quenelles or cold fowls, boiled or roast, with thick cold white sauce or a beef-tea jelly, can be taken when any hot food would create disgust. In cases of violent sickness,

Brand's essence of beef or strong meat jelly can be taken in very small quantities alternately with lumps of ice. Whey is also very useful in sickness, as it can be retained when nothing else can. Unappetising as it looks, people suffering from deadly sickness will keep it down, and it is very nourishing.

For any affection of the bladder the patient will frequently be ordered a milk diet.

The nurse must see the milkman herself and impress on him the importance of sweet fresh milk from one cow being always brought. When brought she must empty the milk into a flat pan, such as is used for rising cream in a dairy; this pan must be placed in a cool place, and must be well scalded each time it is emptied.

The nurse must skim the milk carefully herself, for in such cases the patient must have no cream. The tumbler of milk must be stood in some warm water before it is given to the patient, so that the milk may be of the warmth of new milk. This milk cure is much used and is most valuable, but the nurse must remember that a milk diet is not heating, and that the patient must be kept warm, and great care taken that she should never have a chill while she is undergoing it. The illness itself will conduce to chilliness, and the lowness of diet makes it imperative that the patient should be warmly covered, and that the room be kept of an even temperature.

REMEDIES

AIR AND WATER cushions are of great use to those who have been long in a sick bed. Water cushions are more comfortable and healthier, but they are colder, than air. Each should have flannel and linen cases. A water cushion should be filled with warm water, not hot, but decidedly warm; otherwise it is a most chilling thing. The same rule applies to a water bed. The water in a water bed should be replenished every three weeks; care must be taken to fill both bed and cushions *too* full of air and water. They can easily be reduced when the patient is on them, but cannot be filled, and no one but the patient can tell the exact fulness which is comfortable.

Enemas are constantly given by nurses, but they may be made such a torment to the sufferer that simple as the process is I will write as if the use of them were unknown. When the water is of the right temperature and mixed with the soap, oil, arrowroot, or whatever may have been ordered, the nurse should fill the enema and then empty it once or twice; she should then hold the pipe and tube under the water, while with her hand she firmly squeezes every particle of air out of the enema. She must then withdraw the pressure and let the enema fill gently, touching the bulb to feel that it is well filled, and keeping both tubes and the pipe under water. When the pipe is oiled and placed, the nurse must squeeze the enema steadily, always keeping the other end of the tube under water, so that as the enema is emptied it fills. In this way the patient will have received no wind.

If the patient has suffered much from severe straining, hot flannels applied to the part will be found comforting. At first the flannels must not be applied very hot, as the skin is very tender, but by degrees they may be as hot as the nurse can make them.

When there is illness, whatever the time of year, the nurse should always be allowed easy access to a fire. Hot water, hot flannels, and poultices may be required suddenly in almost every case, and the relief they give is in proportion as they can be applied quickly. A severe headache is often lessened, if not removed, by putting the hands and feet into very hot water. It is a great relief to have the head sponged with almost boiling water; a mustard leaf at the back of the neck is of use in cases of severe nervous headache. When the patient is weary and restless, it will be found soothing to sponge her back and limbs with hot water. Sleep may even be induced, and the nurse can go on sponging while the patient is dozing, never relaxing in the monotonous movement; but she must in such a case have a second person at hand to renew the hot water. If an invalid complains of sudden violent pain in the back or side, the nurse should at once apply poultices and hot fomentations even before the doctor comes. Such pain often means the beginning of internal inflammation, and the hot applications must be used without delay.

The water in which flannels are wrung out for fomenting must be so hot that the nurse cannot bear to put her hands in it; she should, therefore, always have two good sticks about fourteen or eighteen inches long, and several pieces of flannel with hems at each end, into which the sticks can easily pass. The flannels are dipped into water, the nurse holding the sticks, and when the flannel is well soaked she wrings it round the sticks, twisting each way till it is dry enough to apply, when the sticks are quickly slipped out. In this way the flannels are very hot, thoroughly wrung out, and the nurse is not hurt.

Linseed poultices are generally made too hard and dry, and consequently soon become cold and heavy. The nurse should have a basin near the fire into which she puts her linseed, pouring on it boiling water and stirring with a wooden spoon till it is as smooth as cream. The piece of muslin (which is better not quite new) must be at hand, and the linseed poured into it, and the ends turned up over the poultice. A flannel should be laid over the poultice, and sometimes oil silk is used over the flannel, but this makes the poultice heavier. When the poultice is removed, the nurse should wipe, or rather dab, the part with a warm towel, and place a piece of medicated wool where the poultice has been.

Medicated wool, as it is called, is most valuable in cases of rheumatism; it must always be placed near the fire before it is used. When it is warm, it will puff out to double its original size; care must therefore be taken not to put it too close to the fire, or it will be in flames in a second. If liniments are to be used warm, the best way is to place the bottle in hot water. The heating of the liniment causes the stopper to rise, and the bottle is easily upset and its contents lighted if it has been placed by the fire, causing a most alarming aspect of conflagration, although the flame is soon extinguished. In placing the bottle in hot water the label will often come off; different coloured threads should therefore be tied round the necks of the bottles so that the nurse should not make any mistake as to what she uses. Wool sprinkled with laudanum is comforting in cases of acute rheumatism.

Hot bran, or salt bags, give great relief. The bags should be made of flannel and shaped according to the part they are to cover. The bag should not be filled too full. If salt is used it can be heated in the kitchen oven, as it retains the heat. If bran, it must be warmed in a saucepan on a fire in a neighbouring room, as it becomes cold very quickly. While heating the bran the nurse must stir it, and then pour it carefully into the bag, watching that no spark has fallen in. This must be done with the most anxious care, for a tiny spark may easily escape observation, and the bran may be put into the bag with apparently no more smoke than is caused by the heat. Yet after some time the patient finds that her poultice becomes hotter and hotter, and finally discovers that her clothes are smoking, and that they are slowly burning away. In rheumatism of the joints the part affected must be covered with wool, and the wool covered with oil silk. The wool must be constantly renewed, and when taken away it will generally be found to be wringing wet with cold perspiration. Rheumatism often causes intense irritation of the skin, although no eruption or even redness is visible. Boracic acid melted in water will often relieve this, although ointments and soaps have been tried in vain. Most illnesses affect with less or greater importance the water that the patient passes; the nurse should, therefore, have a clean covered utensil in which to keep it, and should never omit to show it to the doctor.

When strapping is required the nurse should be particularly careful only to moisten the ends of the plaster. If, as is often thoughtlessly done, the whole plaster is wetted, it had better be thrown away, as it will do more harm than good. The greatest care should be taken that the lint, or whatever is next to the inflamed part, should protect it well from the plaster. The plaster must be pressed on gently, though firmly, as the surrounding parts of an inflamed spot are sure to be tender. If there

should be any tendency to soreness of skin, the tender part should be washed with brandy and water,
so that the skin may harden; it should always be
most carefully dried. If soreness should actually
exist, or there be anything in the shape of a bed
sore, great comfort will be derived by a small pad
being used. This is merely a bolster of wool covered with linen or washing silk, the ends of which
are sewn together, so that it resembles a giant corn
plaster. The hole must be the size of the sore, the
bolster resting only on healthy skin. It is kept in its
place by straps of plaster placed crossways, the
ends of which are warmed so that they adhere to
the skin. This kind of pad is extremely useful in
the case of boils.

When bandages are required they should be
made of very tightly rolled stuff. Common towels,
if they are smooth, may often be used. They must be
rolled tightly and smoothly, and pinned, so that
when they are required they are fit for use. The
nurse should hold the roll of linen in her left hand,
the end which she has undone being in her right, so
that as she unrolls she tightens. She must fasten her
bandage, if a large one, with safety pins (the American are the best); if a small one, it will be wound

round and across till the limb or joint is well strapped, and can then be sewn.

In cases of advanced cancer, the attendant must remember that the bones are apt to become very brittle. In moving such sufferers the greatest tenderness must be observed. Even with great care a limb will often be broken; and although, where disease has conquered the body so completely, the pain of a fractured limb is small, still the inconvenience and discomfort of a broken limb add to the miseries of the already tormented life.

In moving sufferers the nurse should be very careful to have the night-dress smooth under her arm. A tiny fold of linen may seem perfectly harmless; but if the patient's back is examined after such a tiny fold has been pressed in by the nurse's arm it will be found to be red and indented; the tenderness of the flesh in illness, and the especial sensitiveness in particular cases, cannot be over-estimated.

NERVES

WHEN THERE IS great nervous excitement, the nurse may be able to soothe her patient by holding her hand and talking to her quietly without apparent motive or effort, but keeping her object in view, and becoming gradually silent if she sees that her patient is not becoming soothed.

Nervous people often awake with a sudden start, feeling as if they had been struck violently. It is long before they can become calm, and the startings recur with more or less violence each time they drop asleep. A good remedy for this, if it can be taken, is a breakfast cup of milk in which a tablespoonful of brandy is stirred. This should be taken before the patient settles herself to sleep, and after it has been continued a few nights, the chances are that the nervous startings will have ceased.

Another painful form of nervousness is a convulsive twitch, which patients suffering from nervous exhaustion will often give when wide awake, and which produces a sort of shudder and horror. The nurse may calm much of this nervous condition by gently rubbing the limbs. Rubbing, if skilfully done, will often compose the sufferer and induce sleep. All such rubbings must by done deliberately and with certainty. There must be no *niggling*. The patient must know exactly when and where the nurse's hand will come; she must not rub with jerks and starts, but slowly and smoothly pass the hand up and down. Rubbing is a real art, and, in many cases, a professional rubber will be found to give relief when all other remedies have failed; but all nurses should be able to rub, and to use their fingers, softly and tenderly manipulating the patient. A severe neuralgic headache may be driven away by the slow touch of sympathetic fingers.

The quiet and calm which should make the foundation of a sick-room life are nowhere more necessary than when the patient becomes hysterical.

It is not easy, even with the best intentions, for a nurse to remain perfectly calm with an hysterical patient, and in the effort to do so she often affects either an unnatural gravity or cheerfulness, both of which increase the attack. The nurse should never speak to a person in hysterics, nor look at her. What has to be done in the way of giving salts, cold water, sal volatile, &c., should be done as silently and as naturally as possible. The few words that may have to be said, must be as few and as commonplace as possible. There must be no gaiety and no reproof.

If the nurse feels that there is any danger of her becoming upset herself, she should at once leave the room. A second away, a whiff of salts, will steady her nerves; but if she gives way in the least, her patient's attack will be much more prolonged; and as there is little that can really be done, it will be better that the nurse should remain out of the room. This applies especially to amateur nurses; trained nurses are not liable to be easily affected.

In cases of sore throat, especially if there be any tendency to diphtheria, the nurse must be particularly watchful. The doctor will probably paint the throat with a few drops of muriate of iron mixed with water; but the nurse must not wait for the doctor's visit; she must look down the patient's throat every hour, and if there is the least sign of the fatal white film forming, she must remove it at once with the throat-brush. After having used the brush, she must wash it with the greatest care. The film which has been removed from the throat will stick firmly on to the hairs of the brush, and it must be completely cleared away before the brush is finally rinsed out. Lumps of ice should be given frequently; in such a case the ice acts as a tonic on the throat, and it is an immense boon to the sufferer, whose throat, when in that condition, is most painful.

In cases of severe retching, ice will again be found most useful, and all food should be iced. A lump of ice placed on the nape of the neck will stop the severe straining of sickness. In such cases, when the patient feels inclined to retch, the nurse may stop it by giving her iced water, in which some ozonised water has been mixed, to wash her mouth out with.

Sickness induces great thirst, and, as drinking anything will again produce sickness, the nurse must moisten her patient's lips and even her tongue with lemon juice and water. A patient suffering from nausea should not be allowed to see or smell food, and all handkerchiefs or towels used should be clean. Even when the actual sickness has stopped, it may be brought on again by the sight or smell of anything.

CONCLUSION

IF THE PATIENT should die, the nurse must remember that though her help may still be needed her place is not by the death-bed unless it is requested. She should make her presence felt as little as possible. If she has done her work well in all ways she will find that all turn to her; but she should be perfectly quiet, and forbear to make any remarks or suggestions. Unless she sees that the relations are unwilling to do so, she should make no attempt to close the eyes of the dead nor to tie up the chin.

If all such last duties *are* left to her, she must make her preparations as silently and unobtrusively as possible.

These remarks may seem uncalled for, but experience has taught me that not only the trained but the amateur nurse requires to be reminded that in the presence of death all bustle is unseemly.

To those who have watched and suffered with the sufferer there is nothing but rest at first in the knowledge that death has come, but the feeling of peace is destroyed by the terrible and unreal garb we are in the habit of using for our dead. If instead of the pinked-out band of hard white linen a soft silk handkerchief were placed round the head—if the warm coloured dressing-gown which has been associated with the living might clothe the dead, the last hour would not leave on us the painful impression that it does.

When the requisite washing has been tenderly done, and the fresh white clothes have been put on, the head, bound up by a silk handkerchief, should be laid on a low pillow, not put perfectly flat; the covering, whatever is wished, should be laid over the body, and then the relations, if they have remained away, return, not indeed to find all that they loved, but not to be shocked by a terrible picture which will haunt them long and destroy the memory of what they held most dear.

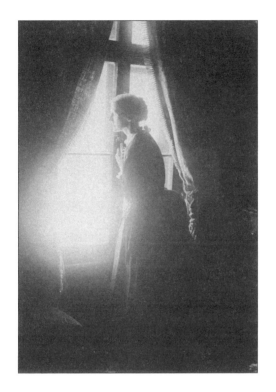

Julia Stephen, 1889.

AFTERWORD

READING ON BEING ILL immediately after reading *Notes from Sick Rooms* reproduces for me, a general internist, the precarious interior balance I try to achieve when seeing patients. I am pretty sure that neither text by itself could have done so. Instead, either one might have thrown its weight behind one extreme or the other of the many polarities that swing through clinical practice, making all the more elusive the necessary equilibrium between knowledge and feeling, the singular and the universal, the private and the public, the embroiled and the safe, and the body and the self that every nurse or doctor or social worker or therapist seeks. But together, these Stephen women wrote me into a shocking recognition of *exactly* what it feels like to be in the presence of a sick person in my care.

We start with the mother. Taking pains to locate the source of her authority in her own clinical experience and astute observation of other experienced nurses, she frames her comments within several governing ideas about "the levelling power" of illness and death, the proportionality between the art of nursing and its resultant pleasure, and the relation of the patient to the nurse not as a personal acquaintance but as a case. With these three conceptual pinions, Stephen commits to a complex description of the ideal nurse, who comprehends and does not fear mortality, derives dividends of joy from the craft of her practice, and develops toward the sick person a posture of engaged concern and educated humility. She is neither smug nor servile, the work on its own neither elevating nor debasing, but, rather, a habit, as Aristotle would have it, of ordinary virtue. Stephen returns to these themes as she closes the essay ("if the patient should die"), taking leave of her reader with the indelible picture of the humble and expert nurse tending the now dead patient with the same equanimity she displayed while the patient lived—no bustle, no fear, no need, no need even to be needed.

The remainder of the essay plunges into the bodily particulars of the sick person. Breezily handling the issue of truth-telling, which continues to bedevil us ethicists (she says "lie freely"), she moves on to the exquisitely sensed corporeal details of being ill. Crumbs in the bed are the most heinous of these insults. Every sense opens the patient to assault, against which the nurse must protect. The smell of the snuffed candle, the too-hot towel after the bath, the too-salty beef tea, the under-filled water cushion, the absence of "gentle hush" in the sick room are examples of the physical torments that cause the patient to suffer. Today, we would call this text "patient-centered," for it depicts the events of illness from the perspective of the patient only. What makes it radically "patient-centered" is that the patient's plight is fully and sensually imagined and privileged. The pappy pillow is felt. The stray hair being dragged across the face with every motion of the hairbrush is felt. The tiny fold in the sheet abrading the skin of the back is felt. The nurse has access to the patient's experience, and it is this access that directs care.

On Being Ill wrenches the reader toward the opposite set of poles. Metaphor trumps matter. The consciousness of the sick person crowds out of sight the corporeal particulars. The flights of passion are reserved not for warm enemas but for the altered mental and creative states accessible through altered physical states. Woolf is concerned with the linguistic and literary aspects of illness more than with the mundane crumbs in the bed—did Proust find the language to describe bodily states is not a question of the state itself but rather of the words available to represent it. The patient crushes together "his pain in one hand, and a lump of pure sound in the other" to produce a brand new word for suffering. This does not have much to do with the smell of snuffed candles but rather with the tropes available to the imagination of that person in pain. It suggests that there may indeed be creative dividends (might this be a desperate hope for a consolation prize?) for the sufferer in the state of being ill. For the mother, the body is the locus of care, and the "mind moves slowly to expression." For the daughter, the body is the transport toward the mind's grasping extremes of meaning, "exalted on a peak and need[ing] no help from man or God."

On one point Woolf is exquisitely clear: there is no such thing as sympathy. "We do not know our own souls, let alone the souls of others." With this, Woolf demolishes the patient-centered stance of her mother. Personal experience is a virgin snowfield crossed by always-first sets of footsteps. "Here we go alone, and like it better so. Always to have sympathy...would be intolerable." Being known, or even accompanied, it seems, would be an intrusion, would cancel out something important about the experience of illness or even about the experience of being.

Mother and daughter disagree about knowability. The mother asserts that the ill person is knowable down to her toes. The able nurse will access the patient's bodily sensations at the very time that that patient undergoes them. She will accurately interpret their meanings and choose proper actions in response. Even the mental states of tension, boredom, and fear are knowable by the nurse. It is for this knowingness that she is trained. The daughter asserts that no one patient is like any other patient. No predictions can be made on the basis of the evidence from others' experience. The experience of illness cannot be generalized. A person is solitary within her illness and, presumably, within her health too. If Stephen's essay ends with a nurse who knows exactly what to do in the face of death, having recognized what is needed both for the dead person and for those who survive the death, Woolf's essay ends with a grief that is not even witnessed. It is not imagined. It is not clucked over. It is noticed by some passing houseguest only by virtue of the hours-long lingering imprint of newly widowed Lady Waterford's agonized grasp on the heavy plush drapes. The widow, and perhaps the author, remain unrecognizable within their grief.

The texts differ not only at the level of argument but also at the level of form. Stephen writes in a diction of tart prescription. "Don't sit on the bed." Generically a rulebook or manual for practitioners, the text gradually produces a righteous voice, asserting the validity of the findings on the basis of her clinical evidence. Woolf from the start uses the improvisational, unrehearsed voice of a searcher, an explorer, one of those brave seamen she reads about in Hakluyt's Elizabethan accounts. The tropes fly a mile a minute; the names of poets and novelists are too numerous to count. Not scholarly, the diction seems a deeply interior one, as if emerging hot off the surface of this one brain.

In both content and form, the two texts seem to me to support radically opposed conceptions of illness, and I think both are required by the effective clinician. I hope to bring to my practice a knowledge born of having watched many persons fall ill and die. I trust that my experience and that of my colleagues point us toward knowing something about what sick people go through. I hope we put that kind of knowledge to use so as to ease the suffering of the patient who comes next into our care. At the same time, I have been humbled by disease. I have come to adopt the stance of radical unknowingness. As long as I don't assume *anything* about a person in my care, I may learn something that will help. No assumptions are justified—on the basis of gender, culture, family, faith, disease, build. Nothing. The more radical my humility, the more I will learn, and the more I can help.

So it is that these two texts come together in this book. So it is that we hope doctors, nurses, social workers, and therapists read them. Like those combination pills that give a patient two medicines adopting two wholly different mechanisms to combat high blood pressure or to lower cholesterol, these two texts do two wholly different things to the clinician-reader to lead to a shared goal. Together, the actions of these two written "interventions" propel the reader toward the clinically powerful stance of radical ignorance, of a recognized engagement with the sick person, of the uneasy truce between freedom and want. Together, these texts supply the contradictory ingredients of the good doctor, the good nurse, the good therapist. Solitary and engaged, imaginative and concrete, humble and flashy, original and tradition-bound, inside and outside: a practical wisdom, Aristotle's *phronesis*, is donated to the sick person side-by-side with a ferocious recognition of the singularity of each experience of sickness or of health.

If you are a patient or if you are caring for a sick person or if you realize that, someday, you and those you love will be sick, you will wish that your doctors and nurses and therapists would have read these texts—together. For together, they catalyze the reader/clinician toward the goal of care—to listen, to recognize, to imagine, to honor.

Rita Charon
July 28, 2012

ABOUT THIS EDITION

THE PARIS PRESS edition of *On Being Ill* closely replicates the 1930 Hogarth Press edition of the book. We selected typefaces that approximate the ones used in the original volume, and the layout closely follows the original design. The front cover includes an original collage by Don Joint, with references to the original 1930 cover art by Vanessa Bell. Inside covers shadow the original 1930 front cover by Vanessa Bell. Vanessa Bell's back cover art now follows the last page of *On Being Ill* in the body of the book. *Notes from Sick Rooms* is added to the first half title page and the title page. A half title page reading *On Being Ill* leads to Hermione Lee's introduction, and another introduces Virginia Woolf's essay. *On Being Ill* is followed by a half title page, *Notes from Sick Rooms*, presenting the introduction by Mark Hussey, and a second half title page that precedes Julia Stephen's Preface and text, followed by a photograph of Julia Stephen, the Afterword by Rita Charon, a note About This Edition, About Paris Press, Biographies, and the colophon.

In ten instances, Paris Press has regularized the spelling and punctuation of *On Being Ill* to conform with the version of the essay that was published in *The Moment and Other Essays* (The Hogarth Press, 1947). The changes include deleting the hyphen in "tooth-ache" (p. 4); using double quotes consistently (pp. 8, 9, 20, 26); inserting a period after "golds" (p.14); correcting the typographical error of "campions" (p. 15); and capitalizing "channel" (p. 24). Paris Press replicated the original use of single quotes throughout *Notes from Sick Rooms*. We also introduced subheads for easier reading, and deleted the running heads that announced different subjects above the text in the 1883 edition. We added an interior photograph of Julia Stephen at the Bear, Grindelwald, Switzerland, silver print by Gabriel Loppe, 1889, reprinted courtesy of the Mortimer Rare Book Room, Smith College. In this new edition, Paris Press corrected four inconsistencies in our first edition of *On Being Ill*, and is grateful to Stephen Barkway and the *Virginia Woolf Bulletin* for pointing them out.

ABOUT PARIS PRESS

PARIS PRESS is a nonprofit literary press publishing overlooked work by groundbreaking women writers and educating the public about these writers and their books through outreach programs. Paris Press values literature that is daring in style and in its courage to speak truthfully about society, culture, history, and the human heart. To publish our books and sponsor educational events, Paris Press relies on support from foundations and individuals. Please help Paris Press keep the voices of essential women writers in print and known. All contributions are tax-deductible. To contact the Press, write to Paris Press, P.O. Box 487, Ashfield, MA 01330, or email info@parispress.org. For additional information about Paris Press, visit www.parispress.org.

Numbered, letterpress, hand-bound limited editions of Virginia Woolf's *On Being Ill* are available for a tax-deductible contribution to Paris Press. Please contact the director at info@parispress.org for specific information.

BIOGRAPHIES

VIRGINIA WOOLF (1882–1941) is among the great literary geniuses of the twentieth century. Her groundbreaking books include *Mrs. Dalloway*, *To the Lighthouse*, *Orlando*, and *A Room of One's Own*. She was an advocate of women's rights, the center of the Bloomsbury Group, and one of the pivotal Modernists. With her husband, Leonard Woolf, she founded and ran The Hogarth Press.

JULIA STEPHEN (1846-1895), Virginia Woolf's mother, grew up in England among painters and poets, novelists and philosophers who frequented the homes of her uncle Henry Thoby Prinsep and her aunt Julia Margaret Cameron, the acclaimed photographer. She worked as a vocational nurse throughout her adult life, and published *Notes from Sick Rooms* in 1883.

HERMIONE LEE is the president of Wolfson College, University of Oxford, England. She is a Fellow of the British Academy, of the Royal Society of Literature, and of the American Academy of Arts and Sciences. She is the author of biographies of Virginia Woolf and Edith Wharton and books on Willa Cather, Elizabeth Bowen, and Philip Roth. Her most recent book is *A Very Short Introduction to "Biography."*

MARK HUSSEY is founding editor of Woolf Studies Annual and has written and edited several books and articles on Virginia Woolf, including *Virginia Woolf A to Z.* He is the general editor of the Harcourt annotated editions of Woolf's works in the U.S., and is on the editorial board of the Cambridge University Press. He teaches at Pace University in New York City.

RITA CHARON is a general internist and literary critic at Columbia University. She directs the Program in Narrative Medicine, where research and training at the boundaries between narrative and medicine occur. She is the author of *Narrative Medicine: Honoring the Stories of Illness* and co-editor of *Stories Matter: The Role of Narrative in Medical Ethics.*

Front cover art and cover design by Don Joint.

On Being Ill text design by Kat Ran Press.

Typesetting for paperback edition of
On Being Ill with *Notes from Sick Rooms*
by Wolf Creek Publishing Services.

Composed in Founder's Caslon and Imprint types.

Interior photograph of Julia Stephen, silver print by
Gabriel Loppe, 1889, reprinted courtesy of the
Mortimer Rare Book Room, Smith College.

Interior art and the inside covers reflecting the original
1930 front cover are by Vanessa Bell and are reprinted
with permission from the Estate of Vanessa Bell.

Back cover photograph of
Julia Stephen with Virginia Woolf,
platinum print by Henry H. H. Cameron, 1884,
reprinted courtesy of
The Mortimer Rare Book Room, Smith College.

Printed by McNaughton & Gunn.